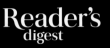

Reader's digest | **Quintessential Guide** to

HEALTHY
EATING

The Truth Behind the Foods We Eat and What to Choose for Optimum Health

....

The Best Advice, Straight to the Point!

D1507495

Reader's
digest

The Reader's Digest Association, Inc., New York, NY/Montreal

A READER'S DIGEST BOOK

Copyright © 2016 The Reader's Digest Association, Inc.

All rights reserved. Unauthorized reproduction, in any manner, is prohibited.

Reader's Digest is a registered trademark of The Reader's Digest Association, Inc.

All illustrations from Shutterstock except p. 15/PhotoObjects.net and p. 16/Getty Images.

Reader's Digest Quintessential Guide to Healthy Eating contains material
first published in *Eat Well, Live Long*.

ISBN 978-1-62145-293-5/Epub ISBN 978-1-62145-294-2

We are committed to both the quality of our products and the service we provide to our customers.
We value your comments, so please feel free to contact us.

    The Reader's Digest Association, Inc.
    Adult Trade Publishing
    4 South Broadway
    White Plains, NY 10601

For more Reader's Digest products and information, visit our website:
    www.rd.com (in the United States)
    www.readersdigest.ca (in Canada)

Printed in China

10 9 8 7 6 5 4 3 2 1

NOTE TO OUR READERS

While the creators of this work have made every effort to be as accurate and up to date as possible, food science and medical knowledge are constantly changing. Readers are advised to consult a qualified nutritionist or medical specialist for individual advice. The writers, researchers, editors, and publishers of this work cannot be held liable for any errors and omissions, or actions that may be taken as a consequence of information contained within this work.

CONTENTS

HEALTHY LIVING

Was there ever a time when food was so readily available and such a source of interest? We should all be terrifically healthy, so what has gone wrong?

Supermarket choice is overwhelming. Restaurants surround us. Food can be bought at pharmacies, gas stations, bookstores, cinemas, department stores—almost anywhere. Cooking shows, glossy magazines, TV advertising, and luscious-looking cookbooks bombard us with images of beautiful meals and extravagant feasts. At the same time, doctors, diet gurus, and government advisers issue dire health warnings about most of the food we eat. It's all so confusing and contradictory.

That is why this book is so important and timely. It is a clear, fresh, and frequently surprising guide to the increasingly complex world of everyday food. It cuts through the clamor of competing interests with one simple message—good, nutritious food is worth seeking out. Why? Because it's delicious, fresh, and made from natural (or near-natural) ingredients, which will promote good health for you and your family. It will make you feel good, help keep you active, combat excess weight, and may also protect you against diseases such as Alzheimer's.

Finding such food should not be a difficult task. Once upon a time, dairy products or meat were procured fresh from their sources; fruits and vegetables came from nearby orchards and farms. But today, when so much of what we eat has been sprayed, processed, frozen, or manipulated in some other way, there is a clear need for expert, unbiased information about what's good for us and what is not—which this guide supplies.

To make this book and achieve that goal, Reader's Digest assembled a team of leading international nutritionists and food writers who understand precisely what goes into modern food products and also how such ingredients influence our health. Now that three-quarters of all food sold across the world is processed rather than fresh, these are vital facts we need to know.

While "processing" can be as minimal as washing leaves or peeling a fruit, it may also strip out nutrients from foods such as grains, while adding any number of preservatives, flavorings, colors, sugar, salt, emulsifiers, gelling agents, thickeners, and more. The added extras disguise the fact that popular "fast" foods—burgers, chicken nuggets, frozen pizza, and pasta dishes—are often made out of "cheap parts or remnants of animal foods," as a 2013 article in the respected medical journal *The Lancet* explained.

The sugar, salt, and fat in these foods appeal to our taste buds; humans are programmed to enjoy—some say even crave—them. In many Western households, ready-made meals and fast foods are the everyday norm. It is a seemingly unstoppable trend that is driving obesity and the global epidemics of diabetes, cancer, stroke, and heart disease, as an increasing number of population studies have revealed. Why? Because fast foods and processed snacks typically supply fattening calories but little fiber and few of the vitamins, minerals, and other important nutrients that contribute to our well-being.

Fighting back against the commercial juggernaut is the most important thing you can do for your own health and the health of your family. The *Reader's Digest Quintessential Guide to Healthy Eating* provides the tools and knowledge to do just that.

WHAT'S HAPPENED TO OUR FOOD?

FOOD, GLORIOUS FOOD!

Most of us live in a world of food abundance. We're not just physically surrounded by the stuff—groaning supermarket shelves, ubiquitous fast-food outlets—but we also face a constant barrage of food ads and cooking programs that stimulate appetites and imaginations. Whether we're hungry or not, there's almost always a tasty snack to tempt us to eat. It's foodie heaven.

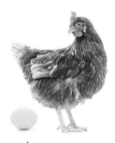

Or Is It? If abundance and availability were all that mattered, we should be healthier than ever, but more and more life-threatening diseases are linked to obesity and to poor diet. In recent decades, choosing what to eat has become increasingly complex.

Once upon a time, all dairy products were fresh from their sources; fruits and vegetables were seasonal and came from nearby orchards and farms. Modern preservation and refrigeration techniques mean that food can be stored longer and travel thousands of miles before it reaches us. So yes, we can enjoy strawberries year-round. But the downside is that much nonseasonal produce has been sprayed, processed, or manipulated in some way before it gets anywhere near a market. A long-distance apple may look red and shiny, but seldom tastes as crisp and sweet or contains as many good nutrients as one just picked from your garden.

Modern processing and mass production have transformed every aspect of everyday eating, filling supermarket shelves with products that were unknown in our grandparents' time. Attractive packaging and advertising persuade us that this or that food product is what we should take home and eat. But all too often, seductively delicious products contain unhealthy levels of salt, sugar, or fats, and few good nutrients.

Faced with the persuasive power of the modern mega-food industry, how do we, as customers, choose food that doesn't just look good but genuinely tastes good and, above all, is good for us? Understanding just what it is you're eating is a twenty-first-century survival skill. Food is at the heart of good health, but, as you'll discover in Part 2, far from sustaining us, some foods and drinks contribute directly to diseases that could shorten our lifespan. Heart disease and many cancers are linked to obesity. And all the evidence suggests that poor dietary choices are primarily to blame for the recent dramatic rise in obesity levels.

Increasingly, too many of us eat processed foods rather than fresh, and although stringent measures have also been introduced in most countries to ensure that foods are safe for consumption, astonishingly, "safe" doesn't necessarily translate to "healthy" or "nutritious." Too often, food products (think anything from chicken nuggets to vegetarian burgers) have become mere industrial widgets manufactured by methods and from a standard of ingredients dictated by profit rather than by health considerations. They won't make you ill because they're moldy or contaminated, but as the 2004 film *Super Size Me* illustrated so well, just thirty days of fast food can have drastic effects on physical and mental well-being.

Processing is not the only issue. It's becoming clear that the intensive, factory-style conditions in which some livestock are raised are not the best for us. Study after study shows that animals that feed or graze in a natural habitat produce tastier, more nutritious meat. Higher-welfare beef has up to 700 percent more beta-carotene than beef from intensively reared cattle, reports Compassion in World Farming. Free-range eggs, for instance, have up to 100 percent more vitamin E and 280 percent more beta-carotene than eggs from caged or battery hens. Similarly, locally grown fruits and vegetables are likely to have lower levels of pesticides and higher vitamin contents than produce transported across the world.

The good news is that you can enjoy good-quality, nutritious, healthy, and tasty food at affordable prices, and this book explains how. In the larger picture, this book embraces and champions the new cultural food revolution that is steadily gathering momentum. Consumer power can be remarkably effective. If more and more people across the world demand better food, the industry that sells to us must respond. The best supermarkets and food manufacturers are already beginning to take heed. Read on . . . and join the revolution!

WE'RE GETTING FATTER—BUT WHO'S TO BLAME?

A third of all Americans are now classified as obese. More than half the population of Europe is overweight or obese, and British obesity levels have—staggeringly—quadrupled in the past twenty-five years, while recent studies show that the problem is spreading through the Middle East and Far East, in countries that have adopted Western-style diets. Medical experts say the situation is reaching epidemic proportions with potentially disastrous consequences. So is self-control—or, rather, the lack of it—really the culprit behind all those expanding waistlines? Have so many of us lost our collective willpower? Or are other factors at work here?

WHY WE LOVE CALORIE-LADEN FOODS

Simple lack of willpower is not a fair explanation, says Dr. David A. Kessler, former commissioner of the U.S. Food and Drug

Administration (FDA). He believes that food companies "addict" us to their processed products with irresistible combinations of fats, sugar, and salt that hoodwink many of us into eating more than we should.

The temptation is compelling because humans are "evolutionarily prepared to respond to fats and sugars," explains Dr. Marc A. Lindberg, a professor of psychology at Marshall University in Huntington, West Virginia, who has studied the U.S. obesity phenomenon for thirty years. We crave these foods because they promote survival. When humans hunted and scavenged for food, high-calorie animal fats were the essential source of energy. Sugars—from fruits and occasionally honey—were rare and highly prized. Much later, says Lindberg, "in a quirk of fate, humans discovered how to take fats and sugars and add them to all sorts of foods to increase production of such foods in homes and restaurants—that's what is responsible for the increases in BMI."

Perhaps the best example of a food that contains both fat and sugar—one you don't need to be hungry to eat—is ice cream. Lindberg offers this example: Given the choice after a big meal, do you want a second helping of the chicken, or the chocolate ice cream? Exactly. The food industry knows this, says Lindberg. It's their business to sell in bulk and make sure we come back for more. Fast foods are engineered specifically to be "addictive"; manufacturers know that people will buy their fatty, sugary, crispy, gooey products because they tap into an evolutionary human response.

MAKING US FEEL PLEASURE

"Addictive" may not be an overstatement, as something else also happens when we munch on chips or bite into a moist piece of cake. Humans are endowed with neural circuitry known as the "brain reward system," which reinforces certain types of behavior by making us feel pleasure. Many researchers believe that food can make this circuitry light up like a pinball machine in an arcade. In fact, studies suggest that the effect of food on the brain could be similar to that of addictive recreational drugs.

Playing a key role in the brain's reward system is a chemical called dopamine. Properly called a neurotransmitter, dopamine affects brain processes that control emotional response, especially the ability to experience pleasure and pain, among other functions. In effect, it triggers your brain to seek rewards, as the release of dopamine makes you feel good. Drugs such as cocaine increase dopamine levels, setting in motion an addictive cycle. Scientists are now discovering that high-sugar and high-fat foods may also overload the brain with dopamine.

In one study, published in the journal U.S. *Obesity* in 2011, researchers at the U.S. Department of Energy's Brookhaven National Laboratory found that the mere sight or smell of favorite foods prompted a surge in dopamine levels in overweight people with compulsive eating disorders. One 2010 study in animals suggested that the same mechanism that promotes drug addiction may be a factor in compulsive-eating behaviors and obesity. Earlier studies involving people of a normal weight found dopamine releases were linked to hunger and a desire for food.

REWIRING **THE BRAIN?**

It was FDA Commissioner Kessler's own lifelong struggle with obesity that prompted him to research the problem, talking to food-industry experts, scientists, and behavior specialists. He also invested hours of his time observing people eating at fast-food joints and restaurants across America. Finally, he concluded why it was so hard for him to control his eating. He deduced that foods that contain fat, sugar, and salt do more than stimulate the brain's reward center. Over time, consuming them actually rewires the brain to the point where the mere smell or sight of such foods activates the reward center, creating the urge to indulge. So you eat, and in response, says Kessler, the brain releases opioids. The result is a pathway in the brain that activates each time you're reminded of those fatty and sugary foods, triggering the urge to eat, whether you're hungry or not. And food companies will do their utmost to make sure that you never forget how delectable their foods taste.

AWARENESS **IS EVERYTHING**

No one is likely to ban the production or promotion of tasty, fattening foods. But making us more aware of them should help. While head of the FDA between 1990 and 1997, Kessler pressed hard for greater accuracy in food labeling. Elsewhere— including Europe, South America, and Asia—similar initiatives have been and are still being launched.

Being aware of the "Big Food" industry's power to seduce you is a vital first step. Knowing that you're being encouraged to eat unhealthy food is half the battle; reading labels is essential, and understanding what your body really needs to grow and thrive repays all the effort. With knowledge comes the power to make better choices. The following pages give you every reason to resist the siren call of food marketers.

Chapter 2

FASTER, CHEAPER . . . BETTER?

In the early days of food processing, innovation was driven by the need to preserve food for leaner times and to make it available to more people. More recently, in a world of huge global food manufacturers, added imperatives are to churn out ever-more products, to encourage greater consumption and boost profits.

The race to produce began in earnest after World War II. Farmers began to use industrially produced fertilizers and pesticides, while subsidies to grow soy and corn encouraged overproduction. The food industry was to find ingenious ways to create a wealth of cheaper fats, sugars, and other ingredients from soy and grains.

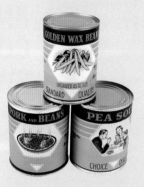

The birth of the tin can

Warfare in the early 1800s prompted the invention of airtight food preservation. When starvation was decimating Napoleon's troops, Nicolas Appert invented a way to seal partially cooked foods in corked bottles, which were then boiled. In 1810, Peter Durand patented a similar method in Britain using tin cans. By 1812, when Britain was at war with the United States, a canned-food factory had opened in London and was soon shipping 18,000 kg (40,000 lbs.) of food a year to the Royal Navy.

CROPS FUEL A FOOD BOOM

Corn and soy oils, for instance, were "hydrogenated," changing their structure to make them more versatile. But the process also created trans fats, now known to be dangerous because they increase the risk of dangerous health conditions, such as heart attack and stroke. The new processed plant oils were originally thought to be healthier than animal fats, however, and advertisers played on their agricultural origins to give them and other grain products a "natural" image.

Soy was processed to make animal feed and various food additives; today processed soy can be found in countless meat-replacement products, such as "veggie burgers" and many other foods. "In fact," writes American good-food advocate and author Michael Pollan in *The Omnivore's Dilemma*, "you would be hard-pressed to find a late-model processed food that isn't made from corn or soybeans."

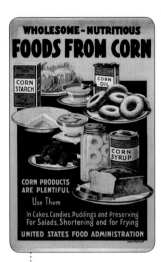

AND A CONTROVERSIAL SWEETENER

Versatile, plentiful, and relatively cheap, these new ingredients proved a boon to the food industry—but potentially disastrous to human health. Sugar, originally derived from sugar cane, was once a luxury reserved for the rich. When Europeans colonized the West Indies and parts of South America, production increased, but it wasn't until the nineteenth and twentieth centuries, when sugar was extracted from beet and other sources, that its use became widespread.

In the United States, a new, cheaper, grain-based source of sweetness was to prove particularly successful. In the 1970s, high-fructose corn syrup (HFCS) was developed. Today, it is present in thousands of foods and drinks, and has been increasingly linked to health problems, even though defenders claim that its chemical structure is identical to other forms of sugar.

The truth is that now most of us consume far too many sweet foods and drinks. With sweetness of some kind added to everything from sauces and pizzas to "healthy" flavored waters, it's almost inescapable. Yet sugar in almost all its forms provides little more than empty calories. Taken to excess, it causes weight gain while offering no nutritional benefits.

CEREAL PRODUCTION— BEHIND THE SCENES

Sugar is one of the main ingredients in many popular breakfast cereals. But there's more to the making of this "healthy" start to the day. The milling process strips away much of the natural goodness of the grain, and what is left of the wheat, corn, rice, or oats is often blended with water into a soupy sort of porridge that goes through an extruder machine. Under high heat and pressure, the mixture is forced out of a little hole, which turns it into its designated shape. For other cereals, grains fed into the extruder expand to become "puffed" cereals. After extrusion, the cereal is sprayed with sugar and oils to help it stay crunchy in milk.

STRIPPED OF ITS GOODNESS

Milling the grain removes the fibrous husks, which contain the nutritionally valuable bounty of fiber, B vitamins, phytochemicals, and some minerals. The heat and pressure during extrusion further destroy the water-soluble B vitamins. Although synthetic vitamins, and sometimes fiber, are often added back into the cereals, the sugar content is often still dangerously high, though many manufacturers have—under government pressure—reduced salt levels in recent years.

But all cereals are not equally bad. Look carefully at your cereal box label. Go for whole-grain cereals, such as breakfast oats, with the minimum of added sugar and salt, and plenty of fiber, which will keep you feeling full. For more information on healthy breakfasts, see page 123.

Chapter 3

FOOD ON TAP

The industrial food revolution that has swept across the world in recent decades has packaged edibles into wonderfully convenient meals and mouthfuls. For many people, cooking is a thing of the past, if indeed they ever learned the skill. For them, preparing a meal now means putting something in the microwave, as ready meals with a range of price tags tempt us to reheat manufacturers' concoctions quickly ("fast" is part of their attraction) rather than toil over a hot stove.

Availability has also turned us into grazers—snacking at home, at our desks, and as we walk or travel—and fast food is the norm for many workers. One 2012 study of 193 schoolchildren aged eleven to fourteen revealed that one in ten of them consumed fast foods every single day and that half bought fast food twice or more times a week. "It is not surprising that . . . many of these children are already overweight or obese and will be likely to become obese as adults," commented the researchers. Globally more than 42 million children under the age of five are overweight or obese—and the World Health Organization blames foods high in sugar and fat.

TEMPTATION 24/7

In towns and cities, the invitation to eat appealing (if unhealthy) food is smack in our faces, 24/7. The eat-me-now aroma wafts over every

Main Street, tempting us with fatty, salty, sugary treats. The two top fast-food chains account for most of the money we spend on fast food, but there are hundreds of other outlets vying to cash in on our appetite for a quick bite.

Fast food is now ubiquitous. You can pick up deli sandwiches, chips, candy, and sodas with your gasoline. Pharmacies, as well as supermarkets, sell take-out foods, often in "meal deals" that actually encourage you to buy a soda and bag of chips along with the sandwich at lunchtime. Shops and stands in train stations sell fast food of all varieties from early morning onward. Vending machines everywhere—even at swimming pools and in sports complexes, which you might expect to promote healthy foods—dispense anything from sweet drinks and chocolate bars to hot pizza and french fries. Cheap, sugary, salty, fatty, unhealthy food is virtually inescapable.

WHY ARE WE DOING THIS TO OURSELVES?

The simple answer is probably because we can. Without giving it a second thought, it is remarkably easy to eat badly and consume many more calories than is good for our health. We eat largely in response to the stimuli around us, says Dr. Brian Wansink, Director of the Cornell Food and Brand Lab at Cornell University.

Most of the time we're surrounded by fatty, salty, sugary foods concocted to appeal to our most basic instincts. Fats gave early humans the energy reserves needed to weather food shortages; the sodium in salt helped them retain water and avoid dehydration; and sugar allowed them to tell the difference between edible berries (sweet) and poisonous ones (bitter), he explains. So, combinations of these ingredients still have the power to hook us.

Making fast food even more irresistible is the fact that manufacturers often price products cheaply and make them supremely easy to obtain. And because it often costs an outlet very little to "supersize" a fast-food meal, we are encouraged to buy the bigger portion because of its perceived value—boosting our calorie intake and the food outlet's profits.

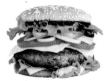

EATING HEALTHILY ON THE RUN

This is not to say that healthy alternatives aren't often sold alongside the unhealthy ones—of course they are. Burger places now sell meal-size salads, for example, and most sandwich shops offer vegetarian choices, whole-grain bread, and low-calorie options. But when you're on the run, you're likely to be under the kind of stress that makes wise choices harder to make, says Dr. Mara Mather, a professor at the University of Southern California Davis, who researches stress and the decision-making process.

"Our research suggests that under stress, the rewarding aspects of an outcome [as in eating a juicy burger] get more attention than the potential negative consequences [as in overloading on salt, fat, and calories]," says Mather. "Even if you do make the apparently healthy choice, you must beware: if you're not careful, add-ons and dressings can make salads nearly as fatty and salty as burgers."

Nutrition experts will tell you that the best place to eat is at the family dining table, with a wholesome, home-cooked meal set before you. But for much of the time, for many people, that's simply not feasible. You may have to work, pick up the kids, drop them at whatever their activities happen to be, and by the time you get home, cooking dinner—much less sitting together as a family to eat it—is an unrealistic proposition for at least one and often more nights of the week. But that's actually no reason why you shouldn't try to make healthier choices. Here are a few ideas:

- **Mind your portions**—If you must have fast food, choose the smallest-possible portion to satisfy your craving, never the supersize one—however much of a bargain it appears to be. You can save more than 800 calories. Or, better yet, share a small portion with friends.

- **Choose the most choice**—Opt for fast-food sandwich outlets where you're in charge of choosing the bread (pick a 100 percent whole-grain option), the dressing (a little olive oil, mustard, balsamic vinegar, or lemon juice), and where you can add vegetable fillings. Choose healthier meats such as chicken breast (roasted, not fried) or turkey, and other lean options.

- **Salad on the side, please**—Always order a side salad when you can, and opt for the low-calorie dressing. It will help fill you up and give you an extra portion of essential veggies.

- **Visit your grocer**—If you're taking your children on an outing, stop at the supermarket first for bottled water, cut-up vegetables, hummus, yogurt, and low-fat cheese—even sushi and salads. Your family might appreciate the al fresco picnic, even if you have to eat in the car.

- **Ask them**—WWBE stands for "What would Batman eat?" This simple question encourages children to make healthier fast-food choices, say researchers from Cornell University. When researchers posed the WWBE question, offering children the choice between apple slices or chips, 45 percent chose the apple slices. Substitute your child's favorite superhero if Batman doesn't do the trick.

BACK TO BASICS

Influential chefs who have taken a fresh, healthy food message into schools or campaigned for locally farmed produce, sustainable fishing, and animal welfare have been making their mark as more and more people prefer to buy produce that has been grown close to home.

The benefits are clear. As the Harvard T.H. Chan School of Public Health points out, most of the fruit and vegetable varieties you'll find in supermarkets were chosen primarily for their yield—how much can be harvested per acre, their growth rate, and their ability to withstand long-distance transport. These are not qualities that are principally designed to benefit our health, nor are they any guarantee of good taste. Farmers producing for local markets are more likely to prioritize good nutrition and taste, choosing their varieties accordingly.

Taste is the driving force behind another campaign that has been gathering momentum across the world. Carlo Petrini founded the Slow Food movement in Rome, Italy, in 1986 to promote traditional foods and counter the influence of a newly arrived McDonald's chain at the Spanish Steps. He believes that our taste buds are being numbed by the onslaught of fast and processed foods and wants people to rediscover the delights of fresh, natural, locally grown foods.

Organic is affordable

"There are many ways that people can buy organic on a budget. Buying seasonally, locally, and directly from growers can save people considerable amounts of money on their food bills. We believe it is possible for most of us to shop and cook organically on a budget and without compromising on quality. It might require some creativity and lifestyle changes, but these changes have the potential to leave both people and the planet healthier and happier."
Josh Stride, Soil Association

MAKING OUR VOICES HEARD

Thanks to the increasing muscle of real-food campaigners—and vocal consumer demand—more local and organic produce is being sold by mainstream businesses, including Pret A Manger and even McDonald's, reports Josh Stride, press officer for the Soil Association, which promotes organic food and farming. There are also more online retailers selling organic produce, and community supported agriculture (CSA) programs offering customers a selection of seasonal fresh fruits and vegetables have become popular.

But the global food industry is a huge force to turn around. When hard times hit, there is increasing evidence that "comfort" food, those tempting fats and sugars, are once more threatening to take hold, especially among those with lower incomes.

"Can't afford to go out for a meal? Never mind, you can still spoil yourself," is the seductive message of many of the "treats" we are sold. But it's not what we or our bodies need. Your food choices matter for your health. The changes you make could be life-saving—and the bonus? Enjoying the delicious taste of real, good-quality food.

FIVE FOOD FOES

GETTING OFF THE BAD FOOD ROLLER COASTER

Do you find that the pounds pile on all too easily and keep piling on year after year? If so, you're far from alone. The simplistic view is that if you're overweight, you must be eating too much and doing too little exercise. The truth is more complex than that.

Much of what we eat today—fast foods, cookies, chips, soda—supplies lots of calories without satisfying hunger. Energy soon flags, together with mood, so we eat some more. It doesn't end there; the fatty, sugary, or salt-laden foods so available in our modern world may actually alter body chemistry in ways that make weight gain and other ailments more likely. These changes are not always as visible as excess pounds; people can be a "healthy" weight and still be poorly nourished. A diet that consists mainly of snacks and fast foods undermines the body's immune system.

Most worryingly, eating like this year after year can encourage the onset of serious, debilitating, and life-threatening diseases, including cancer, heart disease, diabetes, osteoporosis, arthritis, and dementia.

ENEMIES OF GOOD HEALTH

As the world's obesity crisis worsens, the damaging role played by the "Five Food Foes" is gradually being revealed.

- **Bad fats**—People have worried for years about the animal fats in meat, cream, and butter, and their potential for clogging our arteries and causing heart disease. But it took a century for the world to recognize that trans fats, found in certain processed hard margarines and oils, are even worse for our health. Some governments have banned them altogether. You'll discover what sorts of foods contain them and why it's best to steer clear of fast fried-food restaurants unless you know that the oil used for cooking is trans-fat free.

- **Dangerous sugars**—In one form or another, sugars turn up in everything from pizzas to low-fat sauces to yogurts, in most cases adding nothing but empty calories. Learn how to track them down under their many pseudonyms. And find out why cutting back on added sugar and eating naturally sweet foods instead can boost health and also help hold back the years.

- **Super-refined foods**—Many of us eat these most of the time. They're the cookies, pies, ready-made meals, processed meats, and cereal products that line supermarket shelves and make their manufacturers a fortune. But, as global experts have made clear, a constant diet of high-fat, high-sugar, low-fiber fast foods is a major driver for serious, life-threatening illnesses.

- **An excess of additives**—These days, you need a chemistry degree to identify all the preservatives, flavorings, colorings, bulking agents, and more that go into everyday products. Are they strictly necessary? What are they all for? And could some of them be affecting our health? You'll learn some label-reading skills to help you identify the ones that are causing controversy.

- **Evil spirits**—The fifth foe is alcohol, when drunk to excess. Encouraged by powerful marketing forces, it's the richer nations who are indulging, young and old alike. In fact, those between fifty-five and seventy are eight times more likely than young people to need hospital treatment as a result of alcohol abuse. The better news is that drinking wine in moderation and following a few simple rules can actually boost heart health.

FIGHTING BACK

You don't have to ban fatty, salty, and sugary foods completely. But if they form a large part of your diet, cutting back on them makes sense. Your body will thank you for the change. First and foremost, food should nourish rather than harm us, and there's a whole world of great tastes to discover and enjoy. As we learn to appreciate the natural flavors of good food, processed convenience products start to lose their appeal.

Chapter 5

BAD FATS

If you've followed food news over the years, you may have found media coverage of fats confusing. Like in a challenging "whodunit," it's been hard to spot the villain, as advice ricochets from "this fat will kill you" to "this fat will save your life" to "this fat, which we used to think was bad for you, is actually quite healthy, and it's OK to eat a little more of it."

It was back in the 1950s when U.S. doctors first branded saturated fat the ultimate baddie, linking high levels of animal fats in food to the nation's clogged arteries and surging levels of heart disease. By the 1970s, this became dogma, and the food industry responded with a powerful and hugely profitable new low-fat, no-fat revolution. Soon supermarkets were packed with low- or no-fat alternatives for everything from cheese to soups.

Yet close examination of low-fat foods revealed that some had more calories than their full-fat counterparts because they contained more sugar. What's more, after twenty years of low-fat living, people weren't getting any healthier; levels of heart disease and obesity were still rising. In a further plot twist, animal fats came back into vogue as people who wanted to lose weight embraced the low-carb, high-protein meat-based diets of rebel doctor Robert Atkins and his successors. Heart doctors were, understandably, shocked and dismayed.

WHAT WE NOW KNOW

The decades-long confusion is not surprising, but a clearer picture has recently emerged. We know that fat is not, in fact, a single entity, but made up of many different fat types, some of which are much better for us than others. Although the jury is still out on a few more obscure fats, most of the rogues and angels have been identified.

What is also clear and important to understand is that some fat in the diet is essential for the development and maintenance of our bodies and brains. But because fat is densely packed with calories, health problems arise when we eat too much of it, especially the wrong kind. The main types of dietary fat are these:

6 SOURCES OF SATURATED FAT

- Fatty cuts of meat
- High-fat cheese
- Cream and whole-fat milk
- Butter
- Dairy ice cream and ice-cream products
- Palm and coconut oil

- Saturated fat

- Trans fat (hydrogenated vegetable oils)

- Polyunsaturated fat

- Monounsaturated fat

- Omega-3 and omega-6 fats

In this section, we put the first two under the microscope: saturated fat, the original culprit, found in animal and dairy products, and the newer, twentieth-century villain, trans fats, which are produced in the manufacture of certain hard margarines and hydrogenated oils. You'll discover why you should limit the former and banish the latter. In Part 3 you will read much more about polyunsaturated and monounsaturated fats and omega-3 and omega-6 fatty acids, including their virtues and the role they all play in a good, healthy diet.

SATURATED FAT

The fat that makes meat, cream, and butter taste so good is saturated fat; the term "saturated" refers to its chemical structure, which is saturated with hydrogen. These fats—often from animal sources—are widely used because they're stable, have a long shelf life and a high melting point.

Eating too much saturated fat—more than the 20 grams to 30 grams a day, nutritionists suggest—may cause weight gain and has been linked to heart disease, stroke, and diabetes. This is because saturated fats raise cholesterol and can make cells resistant to insulin.

In the health story so far, all saturated fat is dubbed "bad," but this does not present the whole picture. This type of fat is made up of several kinds of "fatty acids," found in both animal and non-animal sources. The problem for even the best-informed consumer is that saturated fat is usually made up of both "bad" and "OK" kinds of fatty acids. So what do we do? Since it's almost impossible to cut out saturated fat altogether, the answer is to limit the amount we consume. For most people, a little as part of a healthy, balanced diet is nothing to worry about. Which is good news for those who love tasty food.

6 Ways to Eat Less Saturated Fat

- Trim visible fat off meat before you cook or eat it.

- Avoid meats with a marbled, fatty appearance.

- Remove skin from poultry before cooking (or at least, before eating).

- Roast potatoes in a little canola or olive oil instead of frying them.

- Choose a lower-fat pizza topped with vegetables, fish, or prawns instead of pepperoni or extra cheese.

- Eat fewer (or avoid altogether) full-fat dairy products; drink skim, rather than whole milk, for instance.

TRANS FATS—DUBBED "FRANKENFATS"

When it comes to food, nutrition writers don't usually like to paint anything edible as being completely unhealthy. "Everything in moderation" is the motto. But with trans fats— or "Frankenfats," as some have called them—normal rules may not apply.

Research into the link between trans fats and heart disease began back in the 1950s. But at that time, the American Heart Association had started to focus on the need to reduce saturated fat in the diet. At first, fast-food chains such as McDonald's fried their foods in beef fat, but as warnings about saturated fat gradually condensed into health campaigns, pressure mounted to abandon the practice.

In 1984, most outlets switched to using partially hydrogenated oils for frying; the notion was that these plant-based, albeit lab-transformed, fats would be healthier. In fact, by the mid-1980s, some studies were already indicating that the unnatural trans-fatty acids produced during hydrogenation were potentially harmful. Further research confirmed this in the 1990s, and today trans fats are of great concern to health experts. The U.S. Food and Drug Administration finally instituted a total ban on artificial trans fats, beginning in 2018.

Although a small amount of trans fat occurs naturally in the saturated fat of cow's milk, the trans fats that have been hitting the health headlines are all man-made. These are corn and soy oils that have been chemically altered by a process called hydrogenation. In this process, the oil is heated to a very high temperature, and hydrogen is pumped through it. This changes the way that the hydrogen atoms bind to the carbon atoms in the oil, turning the liquid vegetable oils into solid fats.

For food manufacturers, solid fats have distinct advantages over liquid oils. They are easier to handle and don't become rancid so quickly, so foods made with hydrogenated or partially hydrogenated vegetable oils have a longer shelf life. With these benefits, it's hardly surprising that this seemingly user-friendly fat found its way into practically every corner of the food-processing industry. It became an ingredient in a huge variety of processed foods, from cookies and other baked goods to breakfast cereals and ice cream. The problem, as scientists discovered, is that it turned out to be less friendly to the health of the consumer.

To understand what's so bad about trans fats, it helps to compare them directly to the healthiest types—the essential, polyunsaturated fats omega-3 and omega-6. These fats are "essential" to the normal structure of body cell membranes, says Dr. Alex Richardson, a senior research fellow at the University of Oxford's Centre for Evidence-Based Intervention. They keep the cell membranes fluid and flexible, which is necessary for normal "cell signaling," the intricate, inner communication process that keeps all our body systems functioning properly.

By contrast, trans fats are "twisted" versions of the natural polyunsaturated fats and act in a very different way. "The twisted trans-fat molecules pack closely together in cell membranes," explains Dr. Richardson. "That stiffens them and makes them less flexible, which interferes with normal cell signaling." As a result, eating trans fats increases the risk of a multitude of serious health problems, including higher cholesterol and increased risk of heart attack and stroke, insulin resistance and type 2 diabetes, obesity, and infertility.

Emerging research also suggests that a high level of trans fats may affect brain development and harm mental health. The brain is particularly susceptible because it is largely made up of fat—60 percent of your brain is fatty tissue. When this tissue takes in the "twisted" molecules in trans fats, it tries to use them as it would good fats. The result? According to new studies, people who eat a lot of trans fats may also be at increased risk of depression, aggression, irritability, manic behavior, and Alzheimer's disease.

TO AVOID TRANS FATS

- Do not buy or eat products listing hydrogenated or partially hydrogenated fat or oil on the label.
- Skip fried foods when you eat out unless you're assured they're not fried in partially hydrogenated oil.
- Cook with vegetable oil instead of solid shortening.
- Avoid cakes, pastries, and cookies, unless you're sure that they are free of trans fats.

Chapter 6

DANGEROUS SUGARS

Sugar is a simple form of carbohydrate. Carbohydrates ("carbs" for short) are the sugars, starches, and fibers found in fruits, vegetables, grains, and milk products. Your body converts the starches and sugars in food to glucose, which fuels your brain, central nervous system, and red blood cells. Any excess glucose is stored as glycogen in your liver and muscles, or is converted to body fat. If you eat too many simple carbs, you're likely to gain weight.

"ADDED SUGAR" VERSUS "NATURAL SUGAR"

The "foes" highlighted in this chapter are the sugars added to foods—not those that are contained in whole fruits and vegetables, dairy foods, or grains. When you eat natural, unprocessed foods, you also get vitamins, minerals, fiber, and phytochemicals, which help your body digest those sugars and convert them to energy, supporting your health and vitality.

On the other hand, the sugars added to sweets, carbonated drinks, cakes, and pastries add nothing that benefits your health. Sugary products are more likely to contribute to dental problems and often take the place of more nutritious foods that would otherwise be in your diet. For example, studies show that the more carbonated drinks a person consumes, the less milk he or she drinks. Milk, of course, is packed with calcium, protein, and vitamins, while carbonated drinks are a nutritional black hole.

THE "TOXIC" SIDE OF SUGAR

The omnipresence of sugar has many of us hooked. Our innate taste for it and the allure of many foods that contain it encourage consumption—with consequent adverse effects on health. "Sugar does cause problems that other calories don't," explains Dr. Robert Lustig, a professor of pediatrics at the University of California, San Francisco. Sugar is metabolized in the liver to fat, damaging the liver, causing insulin resistance, driving up blood insulin levels, and contributing to diabetes, hypertension, obesity, heart disease, and stroke.

IS CORN SYRUP THE WORST SUGAR?

Evidence is mounting that one form of sugar may be more dangerous than others: high-fructose corn syrup (HFCS). This sweetener is produced from corn and is much less expensive to produce than sucrose, the traditional sugar derived from sugar cane and sugar beet. Chemically, sucrose, familiar to us all as table sugar, and HFCS are different, and some experts believe they behave differently in the body. One study from Princeton University showed that rats with access to HFCS gained much more weight than rats with access to table sugar, even when they ate the same amount in calories.

Know your sugars.

Sweetness comes in many different guises. If any of the following items are listed on a food label, then the product contains added sugar. Since ingredients are listed by weight on labels, if you see sugars among the first few ingredients, you know that the product contains a substantial amount of sugar.

- Brown sugar
- Cane juice
- Cane syrup
- Confectioner's sugar
- Corn sweetener and corn syrup
- Dextrose
- Fructose
- Fruit-juice concentrates
- Glucose
- Granulated white sugar
- High-fructose corn syrup
- Honey
- Hydrolyzed starch

In 2010, researchers at the University of Colorado wrote that "excess fructose intake should be considered an environmental toxin with major health implications." In 2011, results of a study published in the journal *Metabolism* suggested that drinking HFCS beverages raised both blood pressure and blood-sugar levels higher than did sucrose-sweetened beverages. Research published in *The Journals of Gerontology* in 2010 has also linked excessive fructose intake to dementia. HFCS producers have challenged the findings and are contesting the claims.

A CLEAR MESSAGE

All the evidence suggests that we should consume fewer foods and drinks that contain added sugars, and avoid excessive intake of HFCS. Start cutting down as soon as you can. As your sugar intake goes down, your body will thank you; sweet treats send blood sugar see-sawing, with consequent energy and mood fluctuations. Fruits, fresh or dried, are a much more nutritious source of sweetness, offering vitamins, minerals, and fiber, too. Eat naturally to fuel your body with essential nutrients—and see how much healthier you feel.

SUPER-REFINED . . . BUT FAR FROM CULTIVATED FOODS

You hear about processed or "refined" foods, but what are they? In fact, practically all the foods you buy in the supermarket are in some way or another processed or refined. So much happens to our food from the moment a crop is harvested or an animal is slaughtered to the point it arrives on our plates. Processing ranges from the simplest and most basic actions, such as washing vegetables, to transforming foods via chemical additives and machine processes.

TO PRESERVE AND PROTECT

At the minimal-intervention end of the processing scale are actions that don't substantially change a food's composition or its nutritional value. Apart from washing, these would include peeling (although for many fruits and vegetables, peeling and chopping accelerates the loss of vitamins). Expert freezing, drying, and even fermenting are processes that may preserve many of a food's nutrients. Juicing (when the whole fruit is used, with few additives) is also considered a minimal process. But it does alter the structure and food value of a fruit by removing pulp, which contains fiber and nutrients. Moving further along the processing continuum, some perishable packaged foods may have preservatives added to prevent the growth of pathogens—harmful bacteria or mold—and to prolong shelf life. Other foods are exposed to heat, or even radiation, to kill pathogens. Milk, for example, is heat-pasteurized to kill potentially harmful bacteria.

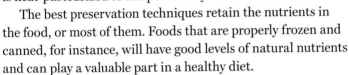

The best preservation techniques retain the nutrients in the food, or most of them. Foods that are properly frozen and canned, for instance, will have good levels of natural nutrients and can play a valuable part in a healthy diet.

TRANSFORMING NATURAL FOODS

Natural ingredients of all kinds are processed and treated to render them longer-lasting and easier to use in fast or packaged food production. When natural ingredients are processed, they often lose their goodness because manufacturing can refine the nutrients right out of them, stripping grains, for instance, of bran, fiber, vitamins, minerals, and phytochemicals to make them easier to package, store, sell, and serve.

A further potentially unhealthy aspect associated with super-refined foods is the manufacturers' tendency to make their products more instantly appealing to consumers by adding the flavors and textures that so many have come to crave (crispy, meaty, gooey, creamy, sweet) via the addition of fats, sugars, salt, artificial colorings, flavorings, and preservatives. This, of course, only encourages us to eat more of certain nutritionally inferior foods.

COMPELLING REASONS TO CHOOSE BETTER

There are many incentives to reach for convenient, often cheaper, fast food. You're busy, perhaps, and time is limited. As you look at the burger, french fries, and soda, you know you're not making the healthiest lunch choice, but how bad for you can a meal like this be just once in a while? A highly refined, fast-food meal now and then won't kill you.

The problem with fast food is not the occasional burger and fries. The trouble starts when such foods are eaten more often. The link between fast foods and obesity is becoming ever clearer. Men who eat fast-food meals twice a week or more are 31 percent more likely than average to be moderately obese, and women with similar habits are 25 percent more likely, according to one study.

CHILDREN AND FAST FOOD

The effect of fast food on children is of particular concern to health experts. While poor diet and inactivity are often blamed in equal measure for obesity in adults, some believe that eating fries, burgers, and high-calorie snacks has a much greater role to play in the worldwide obesity epidemic among the very young.

One long-term study from the UK announced, controversially, that it wasn't lack of exercise that produced fat children. A child's weight gain came first, often in the very earliest years of life. Their data reveals that poor nutrition predisposes a child to obesity and that "portion size, calorie-dense snacks and sugary drinks are all important contributors." Other key findings from this long-term study include:

- Most excess weight is gained before a child ever starts school.

- All children today are at risk, regardless of family income or zip code.

- Parents are often unaware and unconcerned about obesity. Parents can be oblivious to their children's weight, says the study. "Overweight is now perceived as the norm."

We are not designed to consume overly processed foods. Eating fresh, natural produce, cooked at home rather than industrially manufactured, is likely to have a much more positive impact on future health.

GRAIN GOODNESS

The health benefits of eating whole grains—from wheat, oats, and other crops—in bread, muffins, cookies, pasta, breakfast cereals, and more include:

- **Protection against diabetes**—Harvard University researchers found that a diet high in cereal fiber is linked to a lower risk of developing type 2 diabetes, a finding supported by a number of other large, well-conducted studies.

- **A reduced risk of heart disease**—A 2007 analysis of seven major studies showed that people who eat two and a half servings of whole-grain foods a day (compared to those who ate less than two servings a week) have a 21 percent lower risk of developing heart disease.

PROCESSED MEAT AND YOU

Curing meat is an ancient preservation technique dating back to Roman times. Then, the procedure involved little more than salt, smoke, vinegar, and oil. The expensive and marvelous-tasting modern descendants include Italy's *prosciutto di Parma*, Spain's *jamón Serrano*, and France's *jambon de Bayonne*.

When you indulge in such delicacies, you're likely to savor a small amount—because of the price, and also because a little goes a long way. But it's eating processed meats—bacon, sausages, hot dogs, or luncheon meats—frequently and in high quantity that appears to pose the greatest danger. Given what science has told us about the health impact of cured, smoked, and salted meats, you'll be doing yourself—and your family—a favor if you relegate them to the "every now and then" spot reserved for gastronomic indulgences like gourmet ham. One 2010 study from the Harvard School of Public Health found that people who regularly ate processed meats had a 42 percent higher risk of heart disease and a 19 percent higher risk of type 2 diabetes. The World Cancer Research Fund reviewed thousands of clinical studies, and its guidance in a 2012 report was clear: "We advise people worried about cancer risk to avoid processed meat whenever possible."

RED FOR DANGER, OR SOMETHING MORE?

Why is processed meat so bad for us? First, most of it starts as red meat, which has been linked to higher rates of cancer

Key differences

AVERAGE WHITE BREAD V. WHOLE-GRAIN BREAD
(100 g = 4 slices)

2.3 g	Total sugars	2.3 g
44.8 g	Carbohydrate	37.9 g
8.4 g	Protein	9.6 g
2.6 g	Total fat	2.9 g
2.9 g	Fiber (NSP)	6.3 g
127 mg	Potassium (K)	20 mg
29 mg	Magnesium (Mg)	61 mg
86 mg	Phosphorous (P)	146 mg
1.3 mg	Iron (Fe)	2.2 mg
509 mcg	Sodium	486 mcg
0.6 mg	Zinc (Zn)	1.1 mg
28 mcg	Folate	37 mcg

Reader's Digest Quintessential Guide

and heart disease. But it seems that something else is going on, too. Processed meats contain several additives that preserve the meat, including nitrate or nitrite, which forms compounds that are harmful; studies in animals have found they can cause tumors. Many other additives are used during the processing, smoking, or salting of meats that could also promote cancer.

So what should you have in your lunchtime sandwich? If there's leftover chicken from last night's dinner, carve it up and place it between two slices of high-fiber, whole-grain bread, with sliced tomato and lettuce. Buy freshly carved meat from the deli counter, and choose sliced packaged meats—not those described as "re-formed."

CEREAL AND CEREAL BARS

Most breakfast cereals are pretty far removed from natural grains and laced with more sugar, fat, and salt—and far less fiber—than is good for us. What is surprising, however, is that some high-profile cereals specifically marketed as "healthy" are among those high in sugar.

When it comes to cereal bars, matters are even worse. The manufacturers would have you think that these "grab and go" products are perfectly healthy mini-breakfasts that pack the nutritional "oomph" you need to give a good start to your day. They may be called "nutri"-something, or the minimal fruits or nuts they contain may be highlighted to make the product more convincing. However, when a consumer organization's researchers examined thirty different cereal bars in 2012, this is what they found:

- **High sugar levels**—Of the thirty bars examined, sixteen were more than 30 percent sugar. Although in some bars the sugars came from fruit, all but one contained added sugar. One big-brand bar contained 18 grams of sugar per bar— nearly 4 teaspoons.

- **"Trick" labeling**—By law, manufacturers must list ingredients in order of weight. But if a product contains different kinds of sugar, these can be listed separately. This loophole allows manufacturers to list oats, say, higher up the list than the three different kinds of sugar in the product—even though the total sugars may outweigh the oats.

- **Packed with fat**—Ten of the thirty bars were high in saturated fat, including six that were marketed to children. One breakfast nut bar product, labeled "no artificial colors, flavors, or preservatives," contained hydrogenated vegetable oil, which may increase the risk of heart disease. You might think that by putting a cereal bar into your child's lunch box you're giving them a nutrition boost, but in some cases it's just a crunchy candy bar.

BEWARE NOT-SO-HEALTHY "HEALTH FOODS"

Not everything labeled "healthy" actually is. Here are some examples of unhealthy food traps for the unwary.

SMOOTHIES

Nutritionally speaking, these might beat many carbonated drinks, but that doesn't make them all healthy. Smoothies— which come in many varieties—may contain some crushed fruits and fruit juice, which sounds fine, but fruit juice has none of the important fiber that you get from fresh fruits. And if you sip juicy smoothies slowly over time, the acidic juice can damage your tooth enamel. Some smoothies are highly calorific and may contain syrups, sugar, and even peanut butter and chocolate.

TRY THIS INSTEAD: When buying a ready-made smoothie, make sure it contains whole fruit, not just juice. Better still, make your own: in a blender, whizz together fresh fruits and unsweetened, low-fat yogurt.

VEGETABLE CHIPS

You think you're sneaking in a tasty serving of veggies by choosing these instead of potato chips, but you're not. Instead, you're getting lots of calories and fat.

TRY THIS INSTEAD: Air-popped popcorn or a packet of freeze-dried real veggies—just beware of added fat or salt.

BRAN MUFFINS

Anything labeled "bran" sounds as if it must be good for you, because it has plenty of fiber. Not true. Mega-size bran muffins can also have plenty of fat, sugar, and calories, and often contain more than two servings.

TRY THIS INSTEAD: Keep to small bran muffins, or better still, enjoy a bowl of bran cereal with low-fat milk and fresh fruits instead.

FLAVORED VITAMIN AND MINERAL WATERS

Plain old H_2O has become another hot commodity these days, and added vitamins, minerals, or caffeine make it seem as if you're getting something extra for your money. But why pay extra for stuff that you don't need? Some of the enhanced waters on the market are also laced with sugar, so read labels carefully. Similarly, so-called "natural" flavorings in mineral waters with fewer ingredients contain flavoring and up to 6 teaspoons of sugar.

TRY THIS INSTEAD: Tap water that's been chilled in the fridge with a large slice of lemon in it.

GRANOLA

Granola is often fiber-rich and low on the glycemic index, so it keeps you feeling full for longer. It may also contain omega-3 and omega-6 fatty acids, B vitamins, iron, and folate from the rolled oats, fruits, nuts, and seeds. On the down side, many

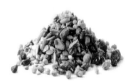

granolas are high in sugar, with more than 12.5 grams per 100 grams; high in saturated fat (5 grams per 100 grams); and high in fat (20 grams per 100 grams).

TRY THIS INSTEAD: Sprinkle nuts, seeds, or fruits over your oatmeal to get the same taste and nutrition as granola, and you'll slash your sugar and fat intake. Or make your own granola by mixing together dried fruits, nuts, a little honey, and canola oil, and pouring this over rolled oats, then baking it in the oven.

FROZEN YOGURT

You avoid the ice cream in the frozen-foods section, going for frozen yogurt as a leaner, healthier option. But is it? Some versions are packed with sugar, so your best bet is to scrutinize the labels before you buy.

TRY THIS INSTEAD: Low-fat Greek yogurt, with live active cultures, is a good alternative here.

WRAP SANDWICHES

Substituting a thin-looking wrap for a traditional bread sandwich might seem a skinnier option, but it's not. The tortilla wrap alone can sneak in as many as 300 to 400 calories, and that's not counting the filling.

TRY THIS INSTEAD: Opt for a sandwich made with whole-grain bread (the grainier the better) spread with a little low-fat mayonnaise, then filled with hard-boiled egg, roast turkey, or chicken, plus a pile of tomatoes, roasted peppers, and dark-green lettuce.

AN EXCESS OF ADDITIVES

Adding condiments to food is nothing new. In early human society, spices were used mostly to preserve food. Today, a vast array of spices is readily available and used imaginatively by amateur cooks and professional chefs. But within food manufacturing, flavor and food preservation are usually achieved in a rather different way.

We take it on trust that food ingredients are good for us—after all, the industry is properly governed and regulated, isn't it? The answer is yes, and sometimes no. And while most of what is added is technically "safe," the other question is, are all these additional extras strictly necessary or conducive to good health?

SALT—NATURAL BUT MISUSED

It is one of the oldest of preservatives—and today the most widely used additive in processed foods. What makes salt so popular in the industry is its capacity for enhancing flavors. Research suggests that at least 75 percent of our salt intake comes from restaurant and processed foods. Salt adds the edge, encouraging us to eat and drink more. Most of us consume more than the recommended maximum of 5 to 6 grams of salt (1.5 to 2.4 grams of sodium) daily.

Why does this matter? Research worldwide has linked a high salt intake to high blood pressure, a dangerous risk factor for heart disease and stroke. Health authorities including the World Health Organization say that millions of premature deaths could be avoided if we all cut back and food manufacturers reduced the sodium content of their foods.

How much is too much in processed foods? Ideally, look for foods with less than 120 milligrams per serving. More than 600 milligrams sodium per 100 grams is "high." Low-salt foods have 100 milligrams of sodium or less per 100 grams. And try not to add extra salt to food; you'll find you soon lose the taste. Instead, use more spices and aromatic herbs to flavor dishes.

FROM CONDIMENTS TO CHEMICALS

What about other food additives—the vast array of chemicals we see listed on food labels? Some are natural, extracted from those once-exotic spices—such as the coloring curcumin from turmeric—and other plant or animal sources. Most are artificial, either re-creating a natural substance or inspired by chemicals occurring somewhere in nature.

Most of the additives used worldwide have clear and distinct functions. They can be broadly classified into these six main groups.

- Antioxidants help prevent foods from spoiling or going rancid, particularly those prepared with oils or fats, which could include everything from pot pies to mayonnaise. They also help to preserve bakery products, soup mixes, and sauces.

Reader's Digest Quintessential Guide

- Emulsifiers, stabilizers, gelling agents, and thickeners are the various ingredients that keep foods from separating, enable foods to gel, and help add body and thickness.

- Flavor enhancers bring out the flavor of foods without imparting any of their own. Monosodium glutamate (MSG) is one of the best-known additives in packaged foods.

- Food colors are used to add color lost through processing, storage, or seasonal variation, and to make the food conform better to consumer expectations. But—and this is an important "but"—it is illegal to use food colors to disguise inferior quality.

- Preservatives limit the growth of microorganisms, enabling foods to be kept for longer.

- Sweeteners, used alone or with sugar, make foods taste sweeter.

THE PROS AND CONS

It is no exaggeration to say that the modern food industry could not exist without its stock of food additives. Those in favor point out that, without preservatives, for example, many foodstuffs would be far more unsafe than they are and that chemicals in food are used only in minute quantities. Many, such as pectin, have a long history in cooking and are known to be harmless; others, such as ascorbic acid (a form of vitamin C), are actually good for you. Some are even permitted in organic food products.

Critics argue that the food industry uses additives not only for the benefit of customers, but also to increase profits, that there are far more additives (including salt) than are strictly essential in foods, and that minute quantities can build up over the long term, with potentially serious health effects. Certain additives are also the subject of heated controversy because they are suspected of directly provoking allergies or behavioral problems. As such, they have become the subject of ongoing research and a target of good-food campaigners.

CAN ADDITIVES WORSEN BEHAVIORAL PROBLEMS?

For more than thirty-five years, researchers have been trying to establish if there is a connection between certain food additives and children's behavior, specifically Attention Deficit Hyperactivity Disorder (ADHD). Parents who believe that certain additives or foods are exacerbating their children's symptoms should ask their doctor if the child could be tested for hypersensitivities. They could then experiment with an elimination diet that excludes the trigger foods.

The bottom line for any food or additive is that anyone can have an allergic or intolerant reaction to anything, but some of us are more sensitive to additives than others. If you suspect an untoward reaction to colorings, aspartame (an artificial sweetener), MSG, or any other additive or food, the best advice is to read labels carefully and avoid food products that contain them. To check whether your suspicions of a specific ingredient or food are correct, as a first step, allergy experts recommend that you keep a food diary. Then, seek your doctor's advice.

Chapter 9

EVIL SPIRITS?

Drink in the Western world—rather like food—has seldom been so ubiquitous or so readily available. While some governments have restricted advertising in recent years, films, television shows, and general peer pressure perpetuate alcohol's "happy" image. It remains the Western drug of choice—socially acceptable until we drink to excess or become addicted, when it can have a devastating effect on health and individuals' lives. The types of drinking behavior that come with a health warning include drinking outside mealtimes, drinking alone, and so-called "binge drinking."

The numbers affected by alcohol are rising. Contrary to the general perception that hazardous drinking is the province of the young, it is the fifty-five- to seventy-four-year-olds whose alcohol-related problems cost most in terms of health care. The so-called baby boomers are a whopping eight times more likely to need hospital treatment because of alcohol than sixteen- to twenty-four-year-olds. Long-term harms include:

- Depression
- Liver and kidney disease
- High blood pressure
- Cancer
- Acute and chronic pancreatitis
- Stroke
- Heart disease

Alcohol misuse can also be fatal in the short term, and it is here that younger age groups are often most at risk. Sudden death can result from acute alcoholic poisoning, and from accidents while people are intoxicated. Drinking can also harm an unborn child through fetal alcohol syndrome (FAS). Women need to be particularly cautious because alcohol can increase levels of estrogen and other hormones linked to hormone-receptor-positive breast cancer. Another reason drinking can increase breast cancer risk is that it can damage cellular DNA.

BUT AREN'T THERE HEALTH BENEFITS, TOO?

So, after all the warnings, what about the media reports claiming that red wine is good for your heart? Or that it can protect against Alzheimer's disease, or even lessen the risk for type 2 diabetes? Is the alcohol industry making it up? Where's the truth?

The fact is that many reputable studies show a variety of health benefits associated with drinking alcohol in moderation. The American Heart Association (AHA) agrees that strictly moderate drinking can raise levels of "good" HDL cholesterol, lower blood pressure, prevent artery damage caused by "bad" LDL cholesterol, and reduce blood clot formation. The key is "strictly moderate," which the AHA defines as no more than two drinks a day for men and just one for women.

Some people cannot tolerate any alcohol: for people who have suffered any chronic illness, drinking can make matters worse and is something that should be discussed with a doctor. In addition, anyone taking medication should ask his or her doctor whether it is safe to drink alcohol.

TOP TIPS FOR HAPPY DRINKING

If you're in good health, a little alcohol may do no harm. Here are a few guidelines that will help to keep your drinking safe and sociable.

- **Keep alcohol for mealtimes**—Evidence from France and other wine-producing countries clearly shows that drinking alcohol with meals is best.

- **Space your drinks**—Sip slowly, so that you're consuming no more than one or, at the most, two drinks per hour.

- **Never drink on an empty stomach**—When alcohol hits an empty stomach, it is immediately absorbed into the bloodstream before the body has a chance to break it down. Eating before drinking—especially proteins, fats, and whole-grain carbohydrates—slows alcohol absorption.

- **Order on the rocks, not neat**—Warmer drinks are absorbed faster—and, therefore, inebriate more quickly—than colder drinks.

- **Watch your mixers**—Carbonated mixers such as tonic and soda add calories and speed up the absorption of alcohol, so you get tipsier faster.

- **Know your cocktails**—Some contain several shots of spirits. Be sure to ask what's in an unfamiliar drink, and alternate with nonalcoholic "mocktails."

FIVE FOOD FRIENDS

WELCOME TO THE WORLD OF THE DELICIOUS

Think of fresh bread baking, a meaty casserole cooking, or the aroma of freshly brewed coffee. It's not just fast or processed foods that turn us on. There are dozens of irresistible aromas, vibrant and subtle colors, and, above all, delicious flavors and textures in the world of natural foods.

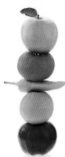

The trick lies in getting to know foods that are quite different from those in the previous section. For every calorie-laden, artery-clogging, blood-sugar-boosting, over-processed, ultra-refined food out there, there is an equally tasty counterpart that will feed your body with the energy and power you need to feel healthy and live longer.

So what is the difference? It's simple, really: the foods described in this section are real foods that remain closer to the way nature made them. To put that another way, they are as "unprocessed" as possible. This doesn't mean you have to raise your own chickens and grow your own potatoes—although more and more people who have the space and inclination are doing just that.

Instead, you'll discover how to navigate the supermarket aisles and explore other food retail options so you can make better, healthier choices for you and your family.

FIVE FRIENDS FOR LIFE

These are the five types of tasty foods and liquids that, in different ways, do the most to nourish your body, safeguard your health, and extend your life by reducing your potential for developing serious diseases.

- **Fresh produce**—The colorful world of fruits and vegetables is perhaps our most important ally against disorders ranging from common infections to diabetes to heart disease. All plant foods (including legumes, nuts, and seeds) are packed with vitamins, minerals, and other micronutrients that keep us in good health. You'll also meet some true superfoods that—without hype—are among the best of the best.

- **Fiber**—It may not sound tasty, but there is plenty to enjoy in this group. Crunchy, whole-grain cereals, grains, nuts, and legumes—plus some of our tastiest fruits and vegetables—are veritable fiber factories that slow the absorption of glucose into your bloodstream and help protect your gut lining against different cancers.

- **Good fats**—Aren't all fats unhealthy and bad for you? Wrong—some, such as delectable olive oil, are actually good for you. Contrary to popular belief, some recent science has proven that adding certain fats to your diet can actually lower cholesterol levels and reduce the risk of a heart attack or stroke.

- **Healthy, lean protein**—This vital nutrient provides the building blocks that form our muscles, bones, and other tissues, and comes in many tasty forms.

- **Water, water, and . . .**—A healthy diet is also about what you drink, and first and foremost among liquids is water.

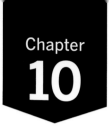

FRESH PRODUCE— NATURAL HEALTH

From the delights of a luscious peach to juicy blueberries, raspberries, and strawberries to ripe, red tomatoes to tender asparagus to leafy green spinach, fruits and vegetables provide an abundance of sensational flavors and colors. But flavor is far from the only reason to enjoy the "five a day" or more that doctors recommend. Never before has there been so much evidence that these foods promote good health. Here are three for starters:

- People who eat the most fruits and vegetables have the lowest risk of developing heart disease.

- Eating plenty of fruits and vegetables may lessen the risk of developing cancer, particularly colon and stomach cancers.

- Those whose diets contain lots of fresh produce have a lower risk of developing type 2 diabetes.

THE KEY TO THEIR PROTECTIVE POWERS

Most fruits and vegetables are excellent sources of multitasking vitamin C. Vitamin C is essential for building teeth and bones, strengthening blood vessels, healing wounds, and creating collagen, the connective tissue that holds cells together and keeps skin smooth.

Vitamin C, together with vitamins A and E, and the mineral selenium are also known antioxidants. They help combat an excess of oxygen-derived "free radicals"—unstable atoms with one or more unpaired electrons. While free radicals fulfill important biological functions, problems arise if our bodies produce too many—often in response to aggravating factors such as smoke, alcohol, or overexposure to ultraviolet light. In a reaction with other molecules called oxidation, free radicals in search of an electron may then oxidize and damage cells, leaving them susceptible to disease.

Scientists believe that is where antioxidants play their vital role, deactivating the oxygen-derived free radicals in various ways before damaging reactions can occur. The table on the following page shows which foods are good antioxidant sources and how much of them we need each day.

FLAVOR, COLOR, AND POWERFUL COMPOUNDS

The slightly bitter taste of cruciferous vegetables, such as brussels sprouts and cabbages, has been linked to a variety of plant compounds (phytochemicals) that are believed to protect against cancer. The vibrant color of many fruits and vegetables is not merely for show. The so-called anthocyanin pigments are often the very components that give fresh produce many of its health-giving properties. That said, plant foods don't have to be highly colored to be rich in beneficial phytochemicals; cauliflower, flax seeds, nuts, and dry beans are all packed with these nutrients. A single serving of most vegetables or fruits will contain hundreds of these potentially disease-fighting substances.

Protective vitamins and minerals in fruits and vegetables

Antioxidants protect the body's cells from damage by free radicals. Vitamin E antioxidant activity also aids immune function and DNA repair. Many fruits and vegetables supply antioxidants—the table below gives a few of the best sources:

VITAMIN/MINERALS	FOUND IN
A	Sweet potatoes, carrots, cantaloupe, pink grapefruit
C	Citrus fruits, strawberries, bell peppers
E	Oils, sunflower seeds, nuts, spinach
Selenium	Brazil nuts, eggs, garlic, and many vegetables

MAKE THE MOST OF FRUITS

Global surveys show that most of us get far fewer than the daily minimum of 400 grams (14 ounces) of fruits and vegetables that the World Health Organization recommends for lifelong health. While children may object to certain vegetables, it doesn't take much to persuade them to eat fruit because it is usually naturally sweet and delicious when properly ripe. You don't have to cook it; fruit could be described as the ultimate convenience food, just needing to be washed or unwrapped before eating. So why do so many of us either fail to buy it or leave it sitting in the fruit bowl until it's only fit to be thrown away?

The trick is to make fresh fruits a habit. Work out how it can best fit into your daily diet, and before you know it, you'll reach your "five a day" and more. It might start at breakfast, with bananas or seasonal berries added to yogurt or cereal. Or a juicy orange could replace an afternoon cuppa and cookie. Or simply take the ten minutes—it's probably no more—to chop up a selection into a fruit salad, and there's dessert. Where possible, buy fruits in season. Take children on outings to pick ripe berries or to help choose them in shops and markets. The more you eat—and the more variety you eat—the greater the health benefits.

SUPERFRUITS THAT NEED NO HYPE

Every so often, little-known fruits will be plucked from obscurity to be acclaimed as bringers of almost miraculous benefits. Think acai berry, pretty mangosteen, or goji berry. Are any of them worth adding to your shopping list? Despite all the promotional hype, the scientific evidence is inconclusive. Studies suggest that more readily available fruits have equal or superior powers. Here is the lowdown on some true superfruits:

- **Apples**—French research reveals that two substances found in apples—boron and phloridzin—may increase bone density and protect against osteoporosis. Other studies suggest that eating apples may greatly reduce the risk of developing cancers of the lung, colon, liver, and breast. Apples also appear to protect against—and reduce the severity of—asthma in children. The pectin in apples may help lower levels of "bad" LDL cholesterol and help control diabetes by reducing the body's need for insulin.

- **Blueberries**—One cup of blueberries supplies 24 percent of daily vitamin C needs and just under 10 percent of your fiber needs, as well as vitamin K and the trace mineral manganese. What's more, a cup of blueberries contains only 85 calories. Blueberries also contain phytochemicals that help decrease the kind of inflammation that leads to chronic diseases. Research has linked eating them to heart, cognitive, and eye-health benefits, while test tube and animal studies suggest they might help fight several different cancers. In fact, all berries—raspberries, blackberries, bilberries, and strawberries—qualify for superfood status.

- **Citrus fruits**—All of these fruits are low in calories and packed with helpful nutrients. UK research in 2011 suggested that the flavanones in citrus fruits may protect against stroke and heart disease. Studies also show that a high intake of citrus fruits can reduce the risk of stomach cancer by 28 percent.

- **Kiwi fruits**—These are one of the most nutritionally powerful fruits. A single large kiwi contains a day's worth of vitamin C, and is one of the few fruits to contain vitamin E. Kiwis also offer fiber and potassium. For easy eating, just cut them in half and scoop out the interior with a spoon.

NUT AND SEED GOODNESS

Nuts and seeds are both delicious to snack on and packed with protective nutrients. Most nuts and seeds are a rich source of B vitamins (such as folate) and vitamin E, as well as minerals including potassium, calcium, and iron. The fats that nuts and seeds contain are the very best kind; walnuts are particularly high in heart-healthy omega-3 fatty acids. Nuts and seeds are a good source of protein, too, and generally high in fiber; several studies have shown that eating them may help to lower "bad" LDL cholesterol. But as nuts are also calorific, it is best to eat no more than one serving a day—about a handful of shelled nuts. Seeds have fewer calories and add variety.

VITAL VEGETABLES

We've probably all come across people who don't like vegetables; the bitter taste of brussels sprouts or cabbage can put children off. The good news is that when vegetables are prepared properly, with flair and imagination, they are delicious—as a main ingredient in meals, for making protein go further, or as side dishes; they are cheap compared to meat or fish.

Perhaps the biggest favor you can do for your health—and your budget—is to learn how to cook with them so that they can become an important, enjoyable part of your everyday diet. To benefit from all their nutrients, as with fruits, you need variety. Here are some vegetable superstars:

- **Alliums (the onion family)**—Onions, garlic, leeks, shallots, and spring onions all contain vitamin C and several B vitamins, as well as important minerals and antioxidant phytochemicals. They also have natural antibiotic qualities that help to reduce inflammation and infection. Cooks celebrate onions and garlic for the flavor they bring to so many dishes.

- **Broccoli**—This vegetable and its cruciferous cousins, such as brussels sprouts and cabbage, are loaded with fiber and good sources of vitamin C and beta-carotene, which the body converts to vitamin A. They may also help protect against cancer.

- **Leafy vegetables**—Superstars kale and spinach may do more than just supply helpful minerals, vitamins, and fiber. The results of a 2010 study suggests that eating 1 ½ extra servings of leafy vegetables a day can reduce the risk of type 2 diabetes by 14 percent. Dark-green, leafy vegetables contain the pigments lutein and zeaxanthin, which, research suggests, protect against cataracts and macular degeneration.

- **Legumes**—Dried or canned, beans (especially red kidney

beans and black beans) pack a powerful combination of nutrients that, among other benefits, encourages healthy sleep and a stable mood. One serving contains as much protein as you'd get from 60 grams (2 ounces) of chicken or fish. They are also rich in fiber; eating them regularly helps to stabilize blood sugar and keeps heart disease and other chronic illnesses at bay.

- **Stalks and stems**—Think asparagus and celery. Asparagus, a late-spring treat, is rich in the B vitamin folate, which helps prevent birth defects. It is also a good source of potassium and many micronutrients, as well as the antioxidant rutin, which is antibacterial and may help to guard against infection. Celery contains folate, vitamin K, and phytochemicals that may help reduce inflammation and fight cancer.

PRODUCE FROM FAR AND NEAR

Few would dispute that a homegrown tomato or an apple from the garden or a local farm often tastes better than a supermarket fruit that has been flown across the world. But is local more nutritious? The answer is, probably. Here are five important facts highlighted by the Harvard T.H. Chan School of Public Health:

- Most varieties of supermarket fruits and vegetables are grown because they produce a good yield and can withstand long-distance transport, rather than for taste or nutrient levels. This also limits our choices.

- So-called climacteric fruits—including apples, melons, and peaches—can ripen after harvesting so are often picked early for long-distance transportation. As a result, their nutrient levels may be lower than those of fruits picked when they are ripe.

- Transporting fruits and vegetables—especially at speed on roads bumpy enough to cause bruising—can further deplete nutrients.

- Cutting, chopping, or slicing long-distance produce to create a "prepared" product can make it more susceptible to microbial spoilage, alter its chemical makeup, and cause it to lose nutrients.

- How fresh produce is stored can also affect its texture, appearance, and flavor.

The reality is that many of us enjoy fruits and vegetables that cannot grow locally or are out of season but available thanks to modern preservation, storage, and transportation techniques. However, as the previous points illustrate, there is every incentive to buy local, seasonal produce when we can—for freshness, nutritional quality, and superior taste.

FIBER—FAR MORE THAN ROUGHAGE

In simple terms, dietary fiber is the edible bits of plants (the cellulose and bran) that resist digestion and absorption in the gut. Most of us know that this substance—also known as "roughage"—is important for keeping constipation and other chronic digestive complaints at bay. It is usually described as having two main components:

- **Insoluble fiber**—Found in whole-grain cereals, bran, brown rice, nuts, seeds, vegetables, and root vegetable skins, insoluble fiber moves through the gut largely unchanged, absorbing up to fifteen times its own weight in water. This helps to bulk up stools and to speed the passage of waste out of your system to prevent constipation and maintain gut health.

- **Soluble fiber**—Found in whole-grain cereals, fruit, beans, and other vegetables, soluble fiber dissolves in water to form a gel-like substance that makes you feel full. By slowing the digestive process, dietary fiber helps regulate blood sugar and insulin levels, reducing the risk of developing type 2 diabetes. It also helps lower "bad" LDL cholesterol levels by binding to excess cholesterol in the gut and by moderating its effects.

DISEASE-FIGHTING **POWERS**

Scientists are now discovering that "soluble" or "insoluble" is not the whole story. What fiber-rich foods do for us is more complex and far reaching than once thought. Certain beneficial effects appear to be due to the way that various components of different fiber-foods interact with the trillions of "good," life-supporting bacteria that live in our gut. Such interactions are thought, for instance, to bolster the immune system, helping our bodies fight disease, and may even improve mood and memory.

What researchers have also discovered is the important role fiber plays in feeding our gut bacteria, giving them a base of support. The best way we can help, they say, is by eating lots of different fiber-rich foods. Just like their human host, it seems our gut microbes need a varied diet that includes a range of fiber components in order to thrive—and when they thrive, so do we. Here are some other findings.

COMBATING CANCER

Researchers have uncovered links between fiber-rich diets and a lower risk of bowel cancer and also oral, larynx, and breast cancers. Bowel or colon cancer is common, especially in the Western world where more processed foods are eaten. One significant finding to emerge from a 2009 study of 520,000 people in ten European countries was that those who ate the most fiber had a 25 percent lower risk of bowel cancer than those who ate lower levels of fiber. The findings also suggested that the protective effect of cereal fiber was stronger than that of fiber from fruits, vegetables, or legumes.

Although scientists have yet to uncover precisely why eating fiber might have a protective effect, what they suspect is:

- When fiber passes through to the large intestine, bacteria there ferment it to produce short-chain fatty acids, which have antitumor properties.

- As fiber speeds the transit of waste through the gut, it shortens the time that potentially cancer-causing toxins are in contact with the gut walls.

- Increasing daily fiber intake means you get more antioxidants, which can prevent the cellular damage that leads to cancer.

BOOSTING HEART HEALTH

Getting plenty of dietary fiber lowers your risk for the whole spectrum of problems collectively known as "heart disease." Recent studies have shown that every 10 grams of additional fiber in your diet can decrease the chances of dying from heart disease by 27 percent. Here are some of the reasons why:

- High cholesterol levels are implicated in more than half of all heart attacks, so it is vital to keep your cholesterol at healthy levels. Soluble fiber works to decrease both total cholesterol and "bad" LDL-cholesterol levels by increasing the rate of bile elimination—out with the bile, out with the cholesterol.

- The short-chain fatty acids produced when fiber ferments in the large intestine during digestion are thought to inhibit the process by which the body makes cholesterol.

- Eating a fiber-rich diet helps maintain a healthy weight, which is one of the keys to keeping heart disease at bay.

- Dietary fiber has anti-inflammatory effects within the body, which may help keep plaque stable so it doesn't break free from blood vessel walls to form blockages within the vessels.

- Fiber might help lower blood pressure and control blood-sugar levels.

PROTECTION FROM DIABETES

Eating a fiber-rich diet helps in two ways: it stabilizes blood-sugar levels, and it satisfies hunger with fewer calories, thus helping control weight. A large study of 42,000 men found that eating fiber from whole grains produced the most significant effect.

Here's how fiber acts: As you digest a carbohydrate, your body turns it into blood glucose, producing a temporary glucose rise before insulin begins to regulate the process. If the food contains fiber, your body has to work harder to break it down and digest it, which slows the rate at which the food is absorbed and converted to blood glucose. This makes it easier for your body to regulate blood-glucose levels and reduces the amount of insulin required to do so.

Eating 25 grams of fiber a day could reduce your risk of developing diabetes by 25 percent. Eating 30 grams of fiber a day has been shown to halve the risk of breast cancer. One reason is that fiber lowers estrogen levels in premenopausal women. Experts believe that lower estrogen levels reduce breast-cancer risk. A second reason is that the higher level of antioxidants that come with eating a fiber-rich diet of fruits, vegetables, and whole grains can help lower cancer risk generally.

SOOTHING DIGESTIVE PROBLEMS

Up to 30 percent of people around the world are affected by various digestive problems, such as irritable bowel syndrome (IBS), constipation, and diarrhea. As different as they are, eating more fiber is often helpful to all of them. A high-fiber diet effectively clears out waste from the digestive system and may reduce the "bloated" feeling that many sufferers experience.

FIBER IN THE FIGHT AGAINST OBESITY

Far wiser than following a low-carbohydrate weight-loss diet is to raise the amount of fiber-rich carbohydrate foods that you eat. People who eat high-fiber diets are generally thinner than those who don't, and they're less likely to put on weight. Here are some reasons why:

Reader's Digest Quintessential Guide

- Fiber-rich foods fill you up and keep you feeling full for longer.

- Fiber-rich foods take longer to chew, slowing down your eating and helping your body to recognize when it's full.

- Weight for weight, high-fiber foods usually have fewer calories than low-fiber foods, so you can eat more of them.

MOOD AND ENERGY

Adding more fiber to your diet may also help you feel less tired. Researchers suspect that one way fiber helps lift mood and energy is that it speeds the removal of toxins from the body.

HOW CAN YOU GET ENOUGH?

You might think that only boring foods are rich in fiber, but nothing could be further from the truth. You get fiber in strawberries, for example, and in grapes and other fruits. As a general guide, about 40 percent of our fiber comes from cereals, 20 percent from vegetables, 13 percent from potatoes, and around 10 percent from fruit and nuts. Some foods supply both kinds of fiber; just as many foods supply more than one vitamin or mineral. Eating a variety of fiber foods is best.

Soluble fiber sources

- Oatmeal
- Oat and wheat cereals
- Lentils
- Apples
- Oranges
- Pears
- Oat bran
- Strawberries
- Nuts
- Flax seeds
- Beans
- Cooked, split, or dried peas
- Blueberries
- Cucumbers
- Celery
- Carrots
- Potatoes

EASY WAYS TO ADD FIBER

If you have a long way to go to reach the recommended fiber intake, don't try to do it all at once. Some people will experience uncomfortable (potentially embarrassing) gassy side effects when they start enriching their diets with extra fiber.

The remedy? Go slowly. One of the best places to start is with breakfast: people who eat high-fiber breakfast cereals are 80 percent more likely to achieve their daily fiber target than those who don't. Then each week, add more servings of fiber-rich foods. Lentils and legumes—such as black beans, kidney beans, and pinto beans—are rich sources, so try lentil soups and bean stews. Fruits like apples and pears are best unpeeled, as they have more fiber with the skin. Get in the habit of reading labels to make sure you are choosing fiber-rich options.

Whenever you're preparing meals, think fiber. Here are eight simple ways to add that little extra into main meals and snacks:

- Add fresh or dried fruits to breakfast cereal—extra points for prunes.

- Replace white pasta with whole-grain varieties.

- Leave skins on potatoes and fruits—that's where much of the fiber is.

- Add chopped raw vegetables to whole-grain pita sandwiches.

- Serve two vegetables and starchy potatoes or grains with dinner.

- Add extra black or red beans—and less meat—when you make chili.

- Add lentils, split peas, or beans to soups.

- Try baked sweet potatoes instead of white potatoes.

Insoluble Fiber Sources

- Whole-grain cereals
- Wheat bran
- Corn bran
- Seeds
- Nuts
- Barley
- Whole-wheat couscous
- Brown rice
- Bulgur wheat
- Zucchini
- Celery
- Broccoli
- Cabbage
- Onion
- Tomatoes
- Carrots
- Cucumbers
- Green beans
- Dark, leafy vegetables
- Raisins
- Grapes
- Fruit
- Skins of root vegetables
- Potatoes

BENEFITS AT EVERY AGE

There are so many delicious ways to include more fiber in your diet—and plenty of incentives. Fiber works at every age. Studies show that mothers who eat plenty of fruits and vegetables tend to have healthier children, who in turn are likely to develop her tastes. Adults will find that including plenty of fresh produce and cereals will help keep them fit and ward off the major diseases described above. And in older age, when you may become less active and when your gut may not function as effectively as it once did, dietary fiber will help relieve constipation and other bowel problems. For good health, giving your diet a fiber boost makes perfect sense.

Chapter 12

GOOD FATS

Given its bad press, you might think that all dietary fat is bad for you. That is far from the truth. In fact, fat, in its many guises, is an essential nutrient that plays a variety of vital, protective roles in your body.

Without fat, we would never survive—or indeed, be born. It's vital from the earliest stages of fetal development. Essential fatty acids, for instance, ensure that our eyes and brains develop as they should. Without fat, you would be unable to absorb vitamins A, D, E, and K, because these need to be dissolved in fat before your body can use them (unlike the water-soluble B vitamins and vitamin C). Fat helps to maintain healthy skin and hair, and supports the body's defenses against harmful viruses and bacteria.

WORKING FOR OUR WELL-BEING

The fats we eat include two—linoleic and linolenic fatty acids—that our bodies need but cannot make. These two fats, found, respectively, in foods such as olive oil and oily fish, help control inflammation, help the blood-clotting process, and are key to brain development. Fatty acids perform some remarkably intricate tasks in the body. They are chemical messengers that trigger reactions controlling growth, immune function, reproduction, and countless other necessary life processes.

Most of these go on inside our bodies without us being even

vaguely aware of them. What can become all too visible, however, are the subcutaneous reserves of fat that insulate the body, keeping it warm and cushioning our internal organs. Dietary fat can all too effectively contribute to this process, piling on excess pounds and endangering our health. That is because fat is such a good energy source: it contains more than twice the calories per gram of protein or carbohydrates. It also makes food taste rich and silky, and transports the fat-soluble compounds that carry flavors—encouraging us to eat.

WHEN "LOW-FAT" WAS GOSPEL

In the past few decades, low-fat diets have enjoyed considerable popularity. Heart-health associations of virtually every country in the world have at some time proclaimed that cutting fat intake in the diet is the key to a healthy heart, as well as the path to slimness.

In the face of this low-fat mandate, food companies created or reworked many products to be low in fat or even fat free, but often adding sugar, salt, refined grains, and other additives to make up for the lost flavor and texture. The result? Millions of people around the world were eating lots of heavily processed foods instead of better, more naturally delicious real foods.

As it turns out, eating just low-fat foods may not make us thinner or healthier. In 2006, results of the eight-year Women's Health Initiative (WHI) Dietary Modification Trial that looked at the health of some 49,000 women revealed a modest reduction in heart-attack and stroke-risk factors, but no reduced risk of heart disease in those who followed low-fat diets. "Just switching to low-fat foods is not likely to yield health benefits in most women," commented Dr. Marcia L. Stefanick, principal investigator of the study.

A BETTER APPROACH

So why didn't the low-fat promise deliver the expected results? One reason is that dieters cut too much fat from their diet, excluding the good as well as the bad, and so lost the health-protection elements that come from fat. Another is that—too often—they replaced the lost fat calories with calories from refined carbohydrates such as white bread, white rice, and potatoes.

Health advice is now clear that some fat belongs in a healthy diet, but too much and the wrong kinds can lead to unwanted weight gain and many other health problems, from heart disease to diabetes. The trans-fatty acids in hydrogenated fats are best cut out of the diet altogether. Saturated fats should be kept to around 11 percent of daily calories—and enjoyed all the more for it. The fats you are about to meet in this chapter are the "good" fats that should form the largest contingent of fat in your diet.

FIND THE FAT

Look at nutrition labels to help you limit the amount of saturated fat you eat.

- **High: more than 5 grams of saturated fat per 100 grams**

- **Low: less than 1.5 grams of saturated fat per 100 grams**

WHAT IS A "GOOD FAT"?

The popular wisdom is that saturated fats, which tend to be solid at room temperature, come primarily from animals, either from meat or from dairy products such as milk, butter, and cheese. Unsaturated fats—often liquid oils—are derived mostly from plant sources, with some from animals, particularly fish. These "good fats" can lower blood cholesterol, ease inflammation, regulate heart rhythms, and much more. There are two types of unsaturated fats: monounsaturated and polyunsaturated.

All the above is broadly true, but the picture is a little more

Food sources of good fats

Cooking oils aren't the only source of healthy dietary fats—some delicious foods are chock-full of them. So what are you waiting for? Here's a guide:

HEALTHY FAT TYPE	FOODS CONTAINING HIGH LEVELS
Monounsaturated	Olives, peanuts, avocados, hazelnuts, pecans, pumpkin seeds, and oily fish
Polyunsaturated	Walnuts, pine nuts, sesame and sunflower seeds, tahini paste, and oily fish
Omega-3	Oily fish—especially salmon, mackerel, herring, and sardines—walnuts, flax seeds, and chia seeds

complex. In fact, even animal fats such as butter and lard contain some mono and polyunsaturated fat, while olive oil and nuts, widely acknowledged to be good for health, contain some saturated fat alongside their impressive quotas of mono- or polyunsaturated fats.

The secret is balance and variety: some saturated fat is important for health, while it is also possible to eat too many "good" fats, as all types of fat are highly calorific. Which is not to downplay their many health benefits when eaten in moderation. This is what they do.

MEET THE MUFAS—MONOUNSATURATED FATS

You'll find MUFAs (monounsaturated fats) in their greatest concentrations in olive, groundnut, and canola oils, as well as in avocados, nuts (almonds, cashews, hazelnuts, peanuts, pecans, and others), and seeds (such as pumpkin and sesame). Making MUFA–rich foods your main source of fat decreases your risk of heart disease and may also help normalize insulin and blood sugar levels.

A key MUFA component is oleic acid (omega-9), which

bestows impressive health benefits on the oils and foods that contain it. For starters, recent scientific research suggests that oleic acid has the power to lower cholesterol, improving the ratio of "good" to "bad" cholesterol, and reduces your risk of heart disease. What's more, it has also been shown to block the action of a cancer-promoting gene called HER-2/neu, which is carried by 30 percent of breast cancer patients. Adding to this beneficial effect is omega-9's apparent ability to enhance the effectiveness of drugs that target that same cancer gene. Olive oil is a particularly good source.

ESSENTIAL FATTY ACIDS—IN NUTS, SEEDS, AND FISH

Polyunsaturated fats (PUFAs) include omega-3 fatty acids, found in greatest concentrations in pine nuts and walnuts, in certain oily fish (sardines, salmon, mackerel, and herring, to name a few), and are also present in various vegetables and fruits, from spinach and kale to avocado and chickpeas. Omega-6 fatty acids are found predominantly in vegetable oils, such as sunflower and safflower, and also in nuts and seeds. Both omega-3 and omega-6 are known as "essential fatty acids" (EFAs) because they're essential for human health—but your body cannot make them, so you need to get them from food. Omega-3 and omega-6 fatty acids are crucial to the growth, development, and function of your brain. They also regulate metabolism, maintain a healthy reproductive system, and keep your skin, hair, and bones healthy.

GETTING THE RATIO RIGHT

Good as both these types of fat are, nutritionists have identified one important problem. Our ancestors ate omega-6 and omega-3 fats in a ratio of 1:1. Because we now consume so many foods that contain vegetable oils rich in omega-6 fats (check labels: they're in many processed foods), the ratio is closer to 15:1, or more. Research suggests that an excessive intake of omega-6 fats may raise the risk of many serious diseases, including heart problems, certain cancers, and autoimmune disorders such as rheumatoid arthritis.

To improve your ratio, cook with olive or canola oils and eat plenty of omega-3-rich fish, such as salmon, mackerel, or sardines.

OLIVE OIL—MAINSTAY OF THE MEDITERRANEAN DIET

The traditional diet of southern Europe is renowned for its heart-healthiness. Study after study support the benefits of eating the way people do in that sun-kissed part of the world. As well as plenty of olive oil, the Mediterranean diet includes lots of vegetables, fruits, legumes, whole grains, nuts, seeds; moderate amounts of dairy, fish, poultry, and wine; small quantities of red meat; and few processed foods.

Golden-green olive oil plays a major role—in both the diet and its benefits. So what makes olive oil so good for us? One

A guide to buying olive oil

- Buy "extra virgin"—This refers to unrefined oil that comes from the first pressing of the olives. It has the freshest flavor and highest levels of phytonutrients, thought to help prevent disease and keep your body working as it should.

- Choose dark bottles—Light and heat can quickly make oils go rancid, so dark bottles are best.

- Seek freshness—The fresher the oil, the higher its content of healthy compounds. Try to find oils that show the date of harvest, or at least a "best before" date.

- Use what you buy—To maintain freshness, buy amounts that you'll use up quickly.

- Experiment—Just like wines, olive oils from different regions vary in flavor, so try them out to find which ones you like best. If you're lucky, you might find a shop that lets you taste different olive oils.

reason is that it's especially high in the key MUFA component oleic acid, which appears to help lower "bad" LDL-cholesterol levels and combat inflammation. It may also help by reducing high blood pressure.

Olive oil is rich, too, in antioxidants called polyphenols. These are the anti-inflammatory compounds that are proven to lower levels of C-reactive protein, the blood measurement used to assess levels of inflammation that indicate the risk of developing heart disease. Polyphenols may also restrict the growth of harmful gut bacteria that cause digestive tract infections.

CANOLA—A HEALTHY COOKING OIL FROM RAPESEED

In about forty years, since commercially viable strains were developed, rapeseed has become the third-largest oil crop in the world. Although now much is used in processed foods, canola oil is firmly in the "good fat" camp. Sixty percent of its fat comes from healthy, monounsaturated oleic acid, and it has the lowest percentage of saturated fat of common cooking oils, at just 7 percent (as compared to olive oil, which contains 14 percent). It is also said to be the most nutritionally balanced cooking oil, with a far lower ratio of omega-6 to omega-3 fats than any other.

Recent Swedish research suggests that the oil may be particularly effective for lowering cholesterol levels. A team from Uppsala University compared the effects of two typically Western-style diets—one containing dairy fat, the other a spread made from canola oil. By the end of the study, the "bad" LDL-cholesterol levels of those on the canola oil diet were 17 percent lower than those on the dairy diet, as were their overall cholesterol levels. Cholesterol-lowering effects of this magnitude are what you might expect to achieve by taking a statin drug.

Chapter 13

HEALTHY, LEAN PROTEIN

Protein is not a single substance. There are at least 10,000 different kinds that play key roles in keeping our bodies working well. Proteins build and repair muscles, skin, bone, hair, and every other body tissue. They make up the enzymes that enable us to digest food, produce the antibodies that fight off infections and disease, and help our muscles move and contract. Proteins transport life-giving substances such as oxygen around the body, and regulate the structure of cells. The list is practically endless.

A VITAL ASSEMBLY LINE

Perhaps the most amazing thing is that your body makes all of these proteins, continually, from protein "building blocks" known as amino acids. Like a great construction engineer, the body follows a "blueprint"—or, to be more precise, a genetic code—to string amino acids together to form different kinds of essential protein.

Scientists have identified more than 150 amino acids, twenty of which are known to be used by the human body. We produce some of these ourselves, but there are nine so-called "indispensable" amino acids that our bodies cannot produce and must be obtained from the foods we eat. Your body cannot store amino acids efficiently in the way it does fats or carbohydrates, so it needs a regular supply.

WHERE DOES PROTEIN COME FROM?

We get our dietary protein from both animal and plant sources, and in two forms. "Complete" protein sources supply all the indispensable amino acids, while "incomplete" sources either lack one or more or don't have them in the right balance. Generally speaking, animal sources supply a complete set of indispensable amino acids, and vegetable sources, an incomplete set.

There are exceptions. Soybeans and quinoa are complete proteins, although both score lower than animal sources on the Protein Digestibility Corrected Amino Acid Score (PDCAAS), used by the World Health Organization to evaluate protein quality. Different plant foods—such as beans and grains—can also be combined to supply a complete source of protein.

So, both animal and plant protein sources provide good matches for our needs, and protein deficiency is rare. But because protein foods come in different packages, what make a difference to our health are the other nutrients each one contains.

MEAT—THE BEST-KNOWN SOURCE

Take, for example, one of the most celebrated forms of animal protein—red meat. A 175-gram (6-ounce) rump steak contains about 40 grams of total protein, or nearly a day's worth. But with it, you also get 19 grams of fat, of which 8 grams is saturated fat. That's around a third of your recommended daily limit for saturated fat (the less-healthy kind), depending on your calorie intake. Compare that to a piece of salmon of the same size, which gives you 35 grams of protein with a similar 19 grams of fat, only 3 grams of which is saturated fat. Then contrast both of these with a cup of cooked lentils with 18 grams of protein yet barely a gram of fat.

This offers a perfect illustration of why it's wise to include lean sources of protein in our diets. No one is suggesting giving up meat; in moderate-size portions, it has much to contribute to a healthy diet. The wisest course of action is to limit portion size, choose leaner cuts of red meat, and not eat it every day.

GRASS FED?

Grass-fed beef is the best option, according to evidence from the Mayo Clinic. Compared to grain-fed beef, it has:

- Less total fat
- More heart-healthy omega-3 fatty acids
- More conjugated linoleic acid, which may protect against heart disease and cancer
- More antioxidant vitamins, including vitamin E

There's plenty of other fresh meat on the menu. Turkey, chicken, and venison all have much lower levels of saturated fats and fewer calories than other meats. Venison is also especially high in protein.

INCREDIBLE EGGS

Eggs are such an excellent all-around source of nutrition that they easily qualify as a superfood. A single egg contains 6 grams of high-quality protein (containing all the amino acids we need), and twelve different vitamins and minerals, including the antioxidant selenium, vitamins B_2 and B_{12}, and the carotenoids lutein and zeaxanthin, which may reduce the risk of macular degeneration, a leading cause of blindness in older people.

Eggs are rich in choline and betaine, two substances that, studies suggest, reduce the "markers of inflammation" in the body linked to chronic health problems, including heart disease, type 2 diabetes, osteoporosis, and Alzheimer's disease. Choline, in particular, plays a role in memory enhancement and brain development.

There is no clear link between eating eggs and the risk of heart disease, as once thought. Most of us no longer need to limit egg consumption, unless advised to do so, as health experts concede that concerns about their effect on cholesterol levels were largely unfounded.

PROTEIN-RICH FISH: THE PROS AND CONS

We're frequently told that eating fish is good for us. Yet, as in so many areas of nutrition today, there's controversy about fish consumption for three key reasons. Some fish contain unhealthy levels of toxins, including mercury, PCBs (polychlorinated biphenyls,) and dioxins. Certain fish, such as salmon, are intensively farmed in crowded pens that can pollute surrounding coastal waters and harm native wild fish populations. Many fish, particularly tuna, have been so overfished that their very existence is in jeopardy.

In 2006, researchers at the Harvard T.H. Chan School of Public Health concluded that eating about 3 ounces of farmed salmon or 6 ounces of fresh mackerel per week reduced the risk of death from coronary artery disease by 36 percent. They also calculated that eating fish regularly reduces premature death from any health-related causes by 17 percent.

Researchers from France delved even further into the risks and benefits of eating fish. They concluded that to benefit most from three key fish nutrients—vitamin D, omega-3s, and the antioxidant selenium—while keeping within limits for potential toxins and minimizing exposure to inorganic arsenic, we should eat a variety of fish in the following quantities: 6 to 8 ounces of oily fish, such as fresh, frozen, or smoked herring; halibut; fresh, frozen, or smoked salmon; swordfish; canned mackerel or sardines; plus 1 to 2 ½ ounces per week of white fish, mollusks, or crustaceans. To minimize exposure to potential toxins, pregnant women can eat most common types of fish, but they should avoid shark, marlin, or swordfish, and might need to limit their consumption of fresh tuna.

ENJOY DAIRY FOODS

Among the most delicious dairy sources of protein are cheese, butter, yogurt, ice cream, and milk. Most are rich in bone-building calcium as well as vitamins A and D. But given that many are also high in fat, can they really play a starring role in eating well and living longer? The answer is yes—in moderation. Here's why.

Together, milk, cheese, and yogurt are relatively low-cost foods that provide a unique package of essential nutrients.

DID YOU KNOW?

"LIVE" BIO-YOGURT IS MUCH HEALTHIER

Yogurt is a top source of calcium, protein, and potassium, but its status as a superfood comes down to the beneficial bacteria called "probiotics," which are present in "live" yogurt. These bacteria help maintain the ideal balance of bacteria in the gut, and we're only just beginning to grasp how important this is for health and longevity. Yogurt with live, active cultures is particularly helpful for people with gut disorders, such as constipation, diarrhea, irritable bowel syndrome, and the *H. pylori* infections that cause ulcers. These beneficial bacteria also enhance immunity. Even people who are lactose-sensitive may be able to tolerate yogurt—so they don't have to miss out on the benefits of this calcium-rich dairy food.

Milk is especially protective. Drinking milk can lessen the chances of dying prematurely from heart disease by 10 to 15 percent and stroke by up to 20 percent. The USDA recommends 3 cups of dairy products a day for most people over the age of eight. Adults and children over the age of five should eat low-fat and skim products whenever possible. Children under twelve months should not have cow's milk, but from one to three years, half a pint of whole milk will supply their daily calcium needs. From ages four to eight years, two to three dairy servings a day is about right. Each of the following counts as one serving:

- 1 cup milk (skim, low-fat, or whole)

- ¾ cup yogurt

- 2 slices hard cheese (cheddar, mozzarella, swiss, Parmesan)

- 120 grams (4¼ ounces) cottage cheese or ricotta cheese

Milk in tea and coffee counts toward an adult's daily intake, as do many other foods such as puddings made with milk, frozen yogurts, or ice cream, and milk-based white or cheese sauces.

WHAT IF I'M VEGETARIAN?

With thoughtful meal planning, vegetarians can get ample amounts of good-quality protein. If you eat them, eggs and dairy products are good sources. Soy foods, nuts, seeds, whole grains, legumes, and lentils also contain plenty; include a variety of them to ensure you meet your protein needs. In fact, a balanced, varied vegetarian diet can be suitable for most people at any age—and can even meet the pressured needs of top athletes. Here are a few examples of important nutrients that plant foods supply:

Soy: much more than a meat substitute

It can seem like the answer to a vegetarian's prayer; soy is not only rich in protein, but also a good source of antioxidants, polyunsaturated fats, B vitamins, and iron. What's more, eating soy can lower your cholesterol and protect the health of your heart. Tofu, a fermented soy food, is a staple of Asian cuisines, which may explain why traditional Asian cultures have lower rates of certain chronic diseases. But in the West, some soy foods (think veggie burgers and nuggets, for example) are highly processed, creating products that are very different from soybeans in their wholefood form. That's why nutritionally minded organizations recommend eating whole soy foods, such as edamame (whole soybeans), and traditionally fermented soy foods such as tofu and tempeh.

- **Calcium**—This nutrient is available in dark-green, leafy vegetables, such as kale and broccoli, baked beans, soy milk, dried figs, and calcium-enriched foods and juices.

- **Iron**—As iron isn't as easily absorbed from plant foods, vegetarians need almost double the iron of meat-eaters. Dried beans, lentils, enriched cereals, broccoli, beetroot, and dried exotic fruits are good sources. Eating vitamin C–rich foods at the same meal enhances the uptake of iron.

- **Omega-3**—If you're not eating fish or eggs, it's difficult to get enough of this essential fatty acid. Soybeans, walnuts, ground flaxseed, and canola oil are sources, and a number of omega-3–fortified products are available.

- **Vitamin B$_{12}$**—If you eat dairy products or eggs, you will get enough B$_{12}$, which is essential for producing red blood cells and preventing anemia. For vegans, sources include yeast extract spreads, fortified soy products, and vitamin-enriched cereals, but supplements may be a good idea.

- **Vitamin D**—Milk and eggs both supply some vitamin D, but the best source of the so-called "sunshine vitamin" is just that—being outdoors in the sun. Vitamin D–enriched cereals, margarine, and soy and rice milks can help those who don't get much sun exposure, or you could take a supplement.

- **Zinc**—This is another nutrient that is not absorbed as easily from plant foods as from animal foods, but zinc can be found in whole grains, soy foods, legumes, nuts, and wheat germ.

WATER, WATER . . . AND A LITTLE WINE

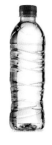

We can survive without food for weeks, but we can't last more than a few days without water. It's vital for health and makes up a surprisingly large proportion of our bodies. A newborn baby is around 75 to 80 percent water, but as we grow and age, the amount of water in our bodies decreases. The total varies from person to person, but, on average, adult men are 60 to 65 percent water, women 55 to 60 percent. Levels also vary between body organs and tissues: the brain, for example, is around 80 percent water, which is why it is so quickly affected by dehydration, while bones are just 10 to 15 percent water. Muscle contains more water than adipose tissue (fat), so in a flabby, obese person, water may be as little as 45 percent of body weight.

HOW MUCH DO I NEED?

Maintaining an adequate amount of water—in other words, keeping your body properly hydrated—helps regulate body temperature and enables your body to dispose of waste efficiently, preventing painful problems such as kidney stones and gallstones. Water is a lubricant that forms the basis of the mucus that lines and protects tissues throughout the body. Pockets of water-based fluid act as shock absorbers for the body's organs, including the brain. In short, water is critical for well-being and healthy growth, with a role in countless biological processes.

A body in perfect balance will take in the amount of water it needs and excrete any excess consumed via sweat, respiration, urine, and feces. On average, adults take in and excrete about 2½ quarts per day. Having a highly efficient water absorption and regulatory system, your body uses water from not only what you drink, but also what you eat, along with a little released from your internal organs. Most people get about a quart a day from food.

So how much should we all be drinking? The guideline amount is about 2 pints a day, or about 6 to 8 glasses; suggestions for as much as 2½ quarts have no scientific basis. The truth is, the amount you need depends on your age, gender, body size, activity level, and a host of other conditions, including altitude and weather. The important thing is to ensure you stay well hydrated—for physical health and to keep your brain sharp and alert.

DOES IT HAVE TO BE WATER?

Milk—an important drink for children—is 88 percent water and, like other drinks (including coffee, fruit juice, and herbal teas), counts toward your recommended daily intake of liquid and may also bring an added bonus in the form of vitamins, trace minerals, or antioxidants. Drinking 3 cups of black tea a day, but no more than 8 cups, could help protect against heart disease and tooth decay.

Coffee, too, has its benefits as a stimulant, but it's not a good idea to drink too much, as it can also have a diuretic effect, increasing the amount of urine you produce. Soft drinks are often high in sugar, and "sugar-free" versions don't necessarily solve this problem, as the sugar is usually replaced by a load of artificial sweeteners. Alcohol is not recommended because it dehydrates rather than hydrates the body.

For all these reasons, most health experts would recommend water above any other drink. Yet there is no scientific evidence to support drinking extra water when you're not thirsty simply to boost health.

BOTTLED VERSUS TAP WATER

With fashionable labels, salubrious sources, and a price point to match, bottled water presents a convincing healthy image. But is it really better than water from our taps? In most developed countries, tap water is perfectly good to drink. It undergoes treatment processes to meet safety and quality standards; some water authorities also add fluoride to reduce the risk of tooth decay.

Bottled water is usually either spring water, which is bottled directly from springs rising from the ground, or mineral water, which also rises from underground but then flows over rocks so it acquires more minerals before bottling. The various brands of both spring and mineral waters contain different types and amounts of minerals, depending on the source.

The bottom line, in the developed world at least, is that tap water is just as good as bottled—possibly better—although the taste may vary from region to region. If you don't like the taste of your local water, try using a water filter, or fill a glass bottle with water from the tap and chill it in the fridge before drinking.

HOW HEALTHY IS FRUIT JUICE?

There is a huge choice of fruit juices on offer—some of them fortified with vitamins and minerals. Nutritionists often

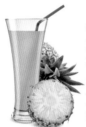

suggest that a glass of juice can even count as one of your five-a-day fruits and vegetables, but be under no illusions. No matter which brand you choose, it will generally contain fewer vitamins, less fiber, fewer phytochemicals, and more sugar than the fresh whole fruit it comes from. Yet juice is undoubtedly tasty and convenient, and healthy enough if the sugar content is not high. For maximum goodness, try the following:

- **Go for whole-fruit juice**—If the juice is made with the whole fruit, the skin included, if appropriate, it will contain more health-giving properties. Shake the container well to disperse any bits of sediment before serving.

- **Go for "100 percent juice"**—You'll know you're not buying added sugar. But check to see if it contains fruits you weren't expecting. More expensive fruits, such as blueberries, may be "stretched" with apple or white grape juice. This isn't always bad: cranberry juice, for example, is so tart it is often mixed with sweeter fruits to reduce the need for extra sugar. Avoid any juice that contains high-fructose corn syrup.

- **Go for natural color**—Juices made from deep purple, red, and blue fruits such as grapes, cranberries, pomegranates, and blueberries are rich in anthocyanins, which are antioxidant and anti-inflammatory.

- **Dilute with water**—adding still or sparkling water to fruit juice creates a more refreshing drink and slashes the sugar content.

WHAT'S SO GOOD ABOUT WINE?

Wine has been part of human culture and celebrations for thousands of years; the New Testament miracle of turning water into wine for a wedding feast illustrates its importance.

In Mediterranean countries especially, dinner without wine is almost unthinkable. Wine, in fact, is one of the elements suspected of contributing to the health and longevity associated with the Mediterranean diet.

The first study to suggest that drinking wine might be linked to a lower risk for heart disease began in Paris in 1967. Called the Paris Prospective Study, it tracked 7,453 middle-aged French police officers over eight years. The results showed that the men in the study, who submitted to medical tests for its duration, had just half the death rate from heart disease as American men—despite the fact that their diet was rich in saturated fats and that many of them smoked.

THE FRENCH PARADOX?

Soon we were calling it the French Paradox—that Frenchmen who enjoyed rich food, wine, and cigarettes had healthier hearts than men elsewhere with supposedly better diets and lifestyles. In 1992, researchers from the French National Institute of Health and Medical Research published the results of a study in *The Lancet* suggesting that the nation's legendary wine consumption had something to do with keeping French hearts ticking. They quoted the findings of other studies showing that 20 to 30 grams of alcohol a day—equivalent to two or three small glasses of wine—could cut the risk of coronary heart disease by 40 percent. Their conclusion was that alcohol seemed to interfere with the clotting ability of blood platelets and that this might be how it helped protect the heart.

Subsequent research reported that moderate drinking of alcohol, not just wine, can lower the risk of heart disease. Research into other potential health benefits suggests it may also improve insulin sensitivity and help combat inflammation.

The key in all of this is the term "moderate." Men and women who drink moderately seem, on average, to gain some benefits over both nondrinkers and heavy drinkers. They are more likely to be a healthy weight, to get the recommended seven to eight hours sleep a night, and to exercise regularly. But imbibe more heavily, and any benefits quickly unravel. When it comes to wine and alcohol, a little is good—but a lot is not. As a general guideline, the World Health Organization suggests no more than two alcoholic drinks a day for women and three for men, with an absolute limit of four drinks on any occasion.

There is a further aspect to the French wine phenomenon. In many cultures, people often drink alcohol on its own and frequently drink to get drunk. But in French and Mediterranean culture, wine is a carefully chosen accompaniment to meals, drunk in moderation to complement flavors and enhance the pleasure of sharing good food with friends and family. That, too, may help to explain its heart-healthy reputation.

IS RED WINE ESPECIALLY HEALTH-BOOSTING?

Probably. Recent research has focused on resveratrol, an antioxidant polyphenol compound present in the skins and seeds of grapes. Red wine has higher levels of resveratrol than white wine because the skins and seeds are left in the wine for longer at the initial crushing and fermenting stage. Resveratrol is the vine's defense mechanism against disease and may also help to protect our health in several ways. ScienceDaily has highlighted resveratrol's potential for "decreasing the body's chronic inflammation response," implicated in many health problems, including heart disease and diabetes. Research at Cornell University suggests the compound may also help decrease plaque formation in the brain, which might protect against dementia.

Chapter 15

ARE YOU MISSING OUT?

Throughout our lives—in fact, even before we are born—the foods we take in affect our health, strength, intelligence, and longevity. The nutrients we humans require are abundantly found in the foods we (should) eat. But to get an adequate supply of those nutrients, we need to choose our foods wisely from the several different food groups and eat them in the proper proportions.

The "Eatwell Plate" can help you consume the right balance of foods necessary for optimal health. This illustration (see next page) makes it simple to picture what should be on our plates—and in what proportions—every day. By following the Eatwell Plate formula, you're likely to get your full complement of vitamins and minerals. But it's good to have a basic understanding of what these essential nutrients are. Let's take a look.

PORTION SIZES

You can scrub your diet free of fast, junk, and processed foods, but you still won't enjoy that zenith of vibrancy or energy if you don't eat food in proper proportions and portion sizes. Dietary balance is key to good health.

The Eatwell Plate

The Eatwell Plate formula illustrates the balance of key types of foods most people should aim for in a healthy diet. Eating these each day in the proportions suggested ensures a regular supply of all essential nutrients.

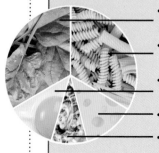

- $\frac{1}{3}$ of your daily diet should be reserved for choices from the fruits and vegetables group.

- another third goes to starchy foods, such as potatoes, bread, and pasta, preferably whole-grain.

- $\frac{1}{6}$ of what you eat should be protein choices from the meats, fish, eggs, and beans group.

- another $\frac{1}{6}$ is occupied by milk and dairy foods.

- a tiny sliver of your daily diet—no more—is the limit for high-fat and sugary foods that you should eat only occasionally.

The best way to achieve that balance is to get to know the number of daily portions you should aim for from the various food categories, which include cereals, breads, meats, fish, grains, dairy, fruits, and vegetables. If you're a normal, moderately active, healthy adult, the following guidelines will ensure you meet your needs for energy and nutrition. If you're overweight, you'll need to trim your portion sizes so that you reduce your energy intake safely, possibly working with a doctor or dietitian. People who are inactive, older, or shorter (especially postmenopausal women) need to eat less food generally, because they have a slower metabolism, which makes it easier to gain weight.

You don't have to stick to single portions of the different foods listed here. What's important is to keep within the suggested daily portion limits. Most people eat much more than they think they do, which is why they put on weight. So keep it real: measure your portions until you have a sense of how much food is appropriate for you.

MEAT, FISH, AND OTHER PROTEINS

3 portions a day. At least one portion a week should be oily fish (salmon, herring, mackerel, sardines). Examples of portion sizes:

- Lean meat = size of a deck of cards/110 grams raw or 65 grams cooked
- Fish = size of a checkbook/115 grams raw or 100 grams cooked
- Eggs = 2 medium
- Baked beans = ½ can/5 tablespoons
- Legumes = 1 heaping handful/4 tablespoons
- Nuts = 1 small handful/2 tablespoons

FRUITS AND VEGETABLES

At least 5 a day, preferably more.

- Mango, pineapple, or papaya = 1 cup diced (or any large fruit)
- Apple, pear, orange, banana, or peach = 1 (or any medium-size fruit)
- Kiwis, plums, or clementines = 2 (or any small fruits)
- Grapes or berries = 1 to 2 handfuls
- Fruit juice or smoothie = 1 small glass
- Peas, carrots, corn, or cabbage, and other vegetables = ½ cup
- Salad greens = 1 cup

GRAINS AND STARCHY FOODS

8 to 10 portions a day. Opt for wholegrain breads, pastas, and cereals. Examples of portion sizes:

- Breakfast cereal = ¼ to ⅔ cup
- Bread = 1 slice
- Potato = ½ baked or 2 small boiled
- Pasta (cooked) = ½ cup
- Rice (cooked) = ½ cup
- Pita bread = ½ round
- Crackers = 3 small

DAIRY

2 or 3 portions a day. Examples of portion sizes:

- Milk = 1 cup
- Yogurt = 1 container (7 ounces)
- Hard cheese = size of a small matchbook/1½ ounces
- Cottage cheese or ricotta = ½ cup

EASY STEPS
TO TRANSFORM
YOUR DIET

HOW TO DO IT

This section is your practical good food guide as you shop, cook, manage your daily meals, grapple with special dietary needs, or embark on weight loss. It is not about rigid formulas or prescriptive meal plans. What is important is to recognize that so much of what is seductively packaged and pitched as "delicious"—think cupcakes, rich ice cream, sugary doughnuts, or sizzling cheeseburgers—is often poor quality and almost certainly not conducive to good health. The challenge is to look beyond profit-making lines to find foods that truly nourish and sustain, and then to ensure they become part of your everyday life.

FIRST STEPS

With food so readily available, it's easy to be "reactive," eating whatever comes our way. The first step is to take control.

- **Getting started**—Here you'll find some home truths about the way many of us now eat and you'll discover fresh incentives to make changes if necessary. You'll also discover what health experts say we should be eating at different times of life, plus tips on keeping track of your diet and some simple ideas for healthy food swaps in everyday meals.

- **Shopping for quality**—Quality food is not necessarily costlier or more time consuming to prepare than less wholesome food. For example, when fruits and vegetables are in season, they are at their best in terms of nutrients and taste, and cheaper, too. You'll discover the best outlets for different foods and how to navigate the confusing minefield of labels and nutrition information on packaged products.

- **Home-made is best**—Cooking doesn't have to take up hours of your time—and it puts you in charge of how much salt, sugar, and fat is in your food. You'll see the benefits of a well-stocked larder and discover plenty of mouth-watering ideas for time and money-saving everyday meals.

THROUGH THE DAY

We need good fuel to function well in our waking hours. Getting the balance of nutrients right helps us feel our best.

- **Breakfast review**—What nutrients does your body need after its overnight fast? The chapter outlines the best breakfast options—including those that take minimal time to prepare—to help you feel alert and keep you going during the morning.

- **Healthy snacks**—Filling up between meals with sweet, salty, or fat-filled snacks can make you pile on the weight, so this chapter looks at *more nutritious ways to* plug the hunger gap.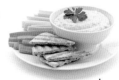

- **Your midday meal**—In today's world, it's easy to rush lunch, postpone it, or even miss it completely. Here you'll find a delicious and versatile selection of healthy options to choose from—including packed lunches—that can all be quickly and easily prepared.

- **Dinnertime**—For many of us, this is the day's key meal. It's often the time when you eat well and relax, share a meal with a friend, sit down with the family, or celebrate a social occasion. This chapter is packed with tasty ideas for preparing quick, nutritious dishes that everyone will enjoy.

TAILORED **TO YOUR NEEDS**

For varying reasons we can't always eat whatever we want to. Here's how to manage different dietary requirements—and enjoy good food.

- **Special diets**—More and more people have to restrict what they eat—often as a result of allergies or intolerances. With a little forethought and planning, most special diets can be easily accommodated with meals that supply all the nutrients required.

- **Effective weight control**—Crash diets are not the answer for people who are overweight or obese. You'll find out how to identify a weight problem and its health implications, how to prepare yourself mentally for change, and where to get the best information. You'll also discover—unsurprisingly—that lifestyle changes, small portions, and balance are among the solutions for long-term success.

Chapter 16

GETTING STARTED

Examining your thoughts about food and eating habits and understanding their significance are vital first steps. But making changes—if you need to do so—should be a gradual process. Your age and current state of health may suggest the sort of tweaks that would help. Start by making small, healthy, day-to-day food swaps, and you'll be much more likely to stick to them, so they will have a bigger, more long-lasting effect.

EAT RIGHT FOR YOUR TIME OF LIFE

Your body has different nutritional needs at different stages of your life. It makes sense, therefore, to tailor your diet to ensure that you meet those needs.

CHILDHOOD

Once weaned, babies need a full range of nutrients in small, easily digestible portions. Also:

- As they grow and get more active, give children vitamin- and mineral-rich cereals and starchy foods, vegetables and fruits, high-protein foods such as poultry, meat, fish, and legumes, and full-fat dairy foods. Give whole milk from the age of one up to the age of five.

- Limit salty, sugary, or fatty foods and carbonated drinks to protect them from becoming overweight and the resulting health problems, including childhood and adult-onset diabetes.

ADOLESCENCE

To fuel their growth spurt at puberty, teenagers need more of most vitamins and minerals. It is now that they lay down stores of minerals such as calcium and iron for later life.

- Energy needs from ages eleven to eighteen increase: a boy's go up by more than 500 calories per day, while a girl's increase by just under 300 calories.

- Growing boys require 13 grams more protein between the ages of eleven and eighteen, while growing girls need around 4 grams more than younger children.

- Three large servings of milk, cheese, and yogurt a day will ensure teenagers get sufficient calcium and phosphorus. They need two or three portions of meat, fish, or alternatives to meet extra iron requirements, plus plenty of fruits, vegetables, and nutrient-dense snacks, such as fortified cereals and bread. Girls also need more iron-rich foods as their menstrual cycle begins.

- As appetite increases at this age, resisting the temptations of fast food is crucial—for good health, and to keep weight under control.

IN YOUR TWENTIES

Studies suggest that this age group eats less healthily than older adults. Some important points to keep in mind:

- Excessive intakes of high-fat, high-sugar, and high-salt foods, plus excessive alcohol consumption, will lead to obesity, raised cholesterol- and blood-pressure levels, and perhaps diabetes.

- Regular exercise several times a week is important now, along with a nutritious diet that includes plenty of calcium (dairy foods, bread, tofu, almonds, and green leafy vegetables) as the body is still building bone. Ensuring you get enough calcium in your twenties helps to combat osteoporosis in later life.

- Women should eat plenty of iron-rich foods such as meat, eggs, dried fruit, green leafy vegetables (for folate, too), and iron-fortified cereals.

DURING PREGNANCY

Pregnant women need foods rich in iron, folate, calcium, and vitamin D, with some vitamin A. (Note, however, that high levels of vitamin A have been associated with birth defects, so avoid liver and supplements.) Expectant moms should eat a variety of starchy foods, fruits, vegetables, legumes, dairy products, lean meats, some oily fish, and well-cooked eggs. Also:

- In the first twelve weeks, a folate supplement is crucial to safeguard the development of the baby's central nervous system and to prevent neural tube defects such as cleft palate, spina bifida, and brain damage. Throughout pregnancy a vitamin D supplement is also advised.

- Getting enough iodine (good sources include sea fish and dairy products) is important as a mild deficiency has been linked to lower IQ levels. By around thirty weeks, pregnant women need an extra 200 calories a day, but "eating for two" is not advised; excessive weight gain (beyond the healthy range of an additional 22 to 28 pounds) can affect the health of mother and unborn child.

IN YOUR THIRTIES AND FORTIES

With career and family responsibilities, activity levels often decrease, while stress and fatigue can prompt poor food choices. Some things to keep in mind:

Reader's Digest Quintessential Guide

- Watch the recommended daily alcohol limit. Too much alcohol can lead to higher blood pressure and weight gain, often at a time when activity levels begin to slow.

- Between the ages of thirty-five and forty, bone mass and density start to decrease. Eating foods rich in vitamin D (eggs, oily fish, butter), calcium (dairy foods and green leafy vegetables), and protein can combat the decline.

- After age forty, type 2 diabetes is more common, too. Risk factors include excess weight, especially around the abdomen. To avoid this and other health problems, eat oily fish, nuts, and beans for protein variety, and get plenty of high-fiber from whole-grain foods. Eating more potassium-rich fruits and vegetables will help combat high blood pressure.

IN YOUR FIFTIES AND EARLY SIXTIES

Both sexes are more susceptible to the cardiovascular damage that cholesterol-clogged arteries can cause. Good nutrition at this time is vital for a healthier old age:

- Be extra vigilant when it comes to salt intake. Excess salt (more than 6 grams a day) is linked to high blood pressure and stroke risk. Cut back on processed foods, which account for 75 percent of total salt intake, and foods high in saturated and trans fats.

- For women, the risk of cardiovascular disease rises sharply after menopause. Muscle mass also decreases, and the loss of estrogen encourages fat deposits—especially around the abdomen. And the rate of bone loss in women accelerates as estrogen levels fall. A healthy diet plus more physical activity will help to counter the natural loss of muscle and bone mass, and control weight, too.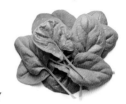

- Eat more "good" fats, whole grains, nuts, and fresh produce, which also supply the antioxidants, B-group vitamins, and polyunsaturated fatty acids identified in a 2012 Polish study as essential factors for maintaining brain health and minimizing the risk of diseases such as Alzheimer's.

AT SIXTY-FIVE AND BEYOND

In older age, both men and women are more vulnerable to infections and other ailments and conditions. Certain nutrients can help:

- Eat plenty of fruits and vegetables for their infection-fighting vitamin C content, to help counter high blood pressure, to control your weight, and to combat diabetes and heart disease.

- Older adults require more vitamin D to strengthen bones against osteoporosis; oily fish and fortified cereals are good food sources. People over sixty-five should also take a vitamin D supplement.

- Eating plenty of fiber, including fresh produce and whole grains, helps combat constipation and digestive problems that often occur in older age.

- Non-starchy vegetables, such as leafy greens, "probably" protect against some cancers of the mouth, throat, voice box, esophagus, and stomach, according to the World Cancer Research Fund and American Institute for Cancer Research. The phytonutrient lycopene, found in tomatoes, may also protect against prostate cancer.

- Older adults should drink 1 to 2 quarts of liquid a day, as thirst decreases but the risk of dehydration, which can cause mental confusion and other physical problems, is higher.

Chapter

17

SHOPPING
FOR QUALITY

If you're short on time and on a tight budget, shopping for healthy food and preparing it might feel like a luxury. But given how important good nutrition is to a long and healthy life—and, conversely, how much damage unhealthy food can cause—it is worth buying and cooking with good-quality ingredients. What many of us forget—as we grab a processed meal—is that you can eat superbly without spending a fortune or half the day in the kitchen.

Many delicious, healthy foods (including eggs, whole grains, and root vegetables) are low priced, while other good but pricier foods can be used in small ways to supplement a dish. Rather than focusing solely on the price tag of food, consider the intangible value of it as well.

This doesn't have to be time consuming. Once you get into the habit of eating healthy, you'll know exactly what you're looking for much of the time. Then you'll be in the best position to resist those alluring snacks and buy-one-get-one-free "bargains."

ASSESSING QUALITY—CONVENIENCE FOODS

Whatever the price, your best guide to the quality of a processed food is the listed ingredients. If you don't want to cut convenience foods out of your diet, select those with:

- Shorter ingredients lists. The ingredients in a food product must be listed by descending order of weight, so anything that appears near the beginning of the list will form a bigger part of the product than those toward the end.

- Few—if any—unfamiliar additives. Although most are safe and some are essential, some you may want to avoid.

EAT WITH THE SEASONS

We've become so used to fresh produce being available year-round in supermarkets that we tend to forget that most fruits and vegetables are seasonal. You should buy seasonally and locally when you can because:

- Produce tends to be fresher because it often comes from closer to home. An expedition to a fruit farm to pick berries can make a memorably delicious and fun family outing.

- Fruits and vegetables are cheapest and tastiest at the peak of their growing season. Some, such as berries, show a definite seasonal curve—not quite sweet enough to start with, rising to a taste peak, then falling off into sourness again. The art is to eat as many as possible when plentiful and at their seasonal best.

- Seasonal fresh produce is likely to be more nutritious. When researchers at Montclair State University in New Jersey compared the vitamin C content of broccoli grown in the United States in season with broccoli imported out of season, they found that the latter had only half the vitamin C. Another study, published in the *Journal of Agricultural and Food Chemistry*, found that the levels of health-promoting anthocyanin pigments increased more than fourfold as blackberries went from underripe to overripe.

- Meat and fish also have seasons, which can affect availability and taste. For instance, spring lamb will have a milder flavor and paler color than the richer-tasting meat from more mature lambs slaughtered in the autumn.

WHY ORGANIC MAY BE BEST

The jury is still out on whether organic foods have measurably more nutrients in terms of vitamins than foods produced by conventional farming, but there is general agreement that organic produce reduces exposure to pesticides, other chemicals, and antibiotic-resistant bacteria.

Antibiotics can only be used to treat cases of illness in organic farm animals; they cannot be used routinely to prevent infection, as commonly happens with factory-farmed animals. Only five pesticides are approved for use on organic crops, and these may only be used in very limited circumstances. By contrast, conventional farmers have more than 300 pesticides at their disposal and use them routinely.

FIVE TOP TIPS

5 tips to make sure you
enjoy good food, even on
a tight budget:

• Buy the best quality
  possible for the foods you
  eat most.

• Save money on basics by
  buying generic, rather than
  branded products.

• Seek out local fresh
  produce whenever possible.

• Buy meat from the butcher
  and fish from a fish seller.

• Exclude all junk foods.

Organic foods rarely contain pesticide residues; whereas, around a third of all conventionally produced food, and almost 40 percent of fruits and vegetables, is contaminated with small traces.

Organic symbols on processed foods flag that the food is less likely to have chemical additives you might wish to avoid. Organic food processors can use only thirty-two additives, and these must come from natural sources, such as vitamin C from lemon juice. So organic versions of processed foods will not contain undesirable additives, such as artificial flavors and colors.

In contrast, 329 chemical additives are permitted in nonorganic food. Some of these are the subject of furious debate on health grounds. No one really knows what the long-term effects of these chemicals on our bodies will be.

THE LANGUAGE OF LABELS

Wherever you're shopping, to be sure that a food is really good, you have to look behind fancy packaging and clever wording to identify the essential facts. Learn to spot the words that may give a product the illusion of being high quality but guarantee no such thing—and make a point of ignoring them.

Many familiar terms seen on food packaging may have no legal definition whatsoever. Watch out for: "artisan," "traditional," "pure," "handmade," "fresh," and "farmhouse." Some products do live up to the promise, but you can't make the assumption without checking the facts. Similarly, a front label may feature mouthwatering pictures of food, or idyllic images of green fields and happy animals. Be sure to read the small-print list of ingredients on the back, which contains the harder facts.

Many food manufacturers are well practiced in strategically placing phrases on their packaging to convince you that the product has a healthy nutritional profile, while distracting your attention from less savory facts. A product with a "low fat" label might sound healthy, but the same product could be loaded with sugar or sodium, which will do you little good.

"No added sugar" sounds promising, but a food or drink with this on the label may contain an artificial sweetener that might be controversial for various health reasons. The phrase "as part of a balanced diet" might suggest that you can eat a product freely, but you need to take its ingredients and calories into account. "Supplies your energy needs" is just a clever way of saying that a food contains calories: it certainly doesn't mean that it's a particularly healthy food.

Finally, remember that a higher price doesn't always equal better taste or quality. If you have any doubts, buy a few different brands, strip off the packaging, and do some blind tasting to test your choices objectively.

THE IMPORTANCE OF FRESHNESS

One of the most important defining characteristics of high-quality food is its freshness. Some foods—such as crackers, chocolate, cereals, dried pasta, and legumes—can be kept for months if stored correctly, usually at room temperature. For more perishable foods—meat, fish, dairy products, eggs, fruits, and vegetables—freshness can be critical. But how fresh is "fresh"? Two labels set out to make it clearer:

- **Use By**—This date label appears on foods that are sold chilled or frozen because they are highly perishable and could give you food poisoning if you eat them after the stated date. Foods that come into this category include chicken, soft cheese, and cooked cold meats. The date assumes that you will store the product according to the instructions on the packaging. Once you open a food with a "Use By" date, you need to follow the instructions on the packaging such as "eat within one day of opening."

- **Best Before**—This date label appears on less-perishable foods, for example, lentils, pasta, rice, and canned tomatoes. When the date has passed, it doesn't mean that the food will poison you if you eat it, but it is an indication that it could be past its prime. For instance, crackers might become a bit soft or stale. Dried fruit might lose its fruity freshness and become hard and sugary. Old legumes might take far longer to soften.

- **Two other date marks**—"Display Until" and "Sell By"—often appear on food packaging. These are not aimed at customers but are instructions for the guidance of market staff to assist stock rotation.

You shouldn't use any food or drink after the "Use By" date, even if it looks and smells fine. You can, however, freeze a food before that date and thereby extend its life quite safely. If you do this, it's important to follow any instructions on the pack, such as "cook from frozen" or "defrost thoroughly before use and use within 24 hours."

While both "Use By" and "Best Before" dates are helpful, bear in mind that there are different types of freshness, too:

- Naturally fresh describes foods—such as fruits and vegetables—that have been recently harvested. There is a relatively short window of opportunity to enjoy them. Usually you will buy/harvest them close to their source and quickly eat them while at their best—a matter of hours, rather than days.

- Stored fresh describes perishable fresh foods that have had their natural shelf life and availability extended by the use of technology. For instance, fresh apples and pears may be picked in autumn and stored at cool temperatures in air modified by removing the oxygen. Then they're sold as fresh produce until the next season's crop arrives. A "stored fresh" apple may be softer, less crunchy, and more "mealy" than the naturally fresh equivalent. Grapes can also have their life extended after picking by being stored and treated with chemical fumigants, such as sulfur dioxide, which can leave a detectable dank smell on them.

- Chilled fresh describes fresh foods sold in chilled display cases. The aura of freshness enables them to sell for more than frozen, canned, or dried equivalents. But it's worth remembering that many chilled products have surprisingly long shelf lives. Milk will often have a "Use By" date for ten days in the future. To extend shelf life, many chilled processed foods may contain chemical preservatives that would not be in naturally fresh food.

- Frozen fresh may have a more down-market image, but when you compare like with like, frozen food tends to have fewer additives than the chilled equivalent. In nutritional terms, there's a strong argument that food frozen when truly fresh— such as freshly picked peas, for example—will be nutritionally superior to a chilled or even fresh equivalent, which may hang around on the shelf for days or even weeks.

- Processed fresh describes chilled, processed convenience foods, such as fruit yogurts, ready-made meals, sandwiches, and desserts. These sell as "fresh," but some of the ingredients may not exactly fit that bill. Eggs in convenience foods are rarely freshly shelled; instead, manufacturers use liquid pasteurized egg, or egg powder reconstituted with water.

Chapter 18

HOMEMADE IS BEST

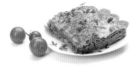

The pressures of modern life can make us feel that cooking is simply too time consuming. As a result, many of us eat out more, and ready-made convenience foods become a larger part of our diet. However much you enjoy a restaurant meal or like the quick option of a ready-made meal or takeout, eating mostly homemade food—freshly cooked from unprocessed, raw ingredients—is by far the better option for your own and your family's health throughout life.

Simple home cooking will almost certainly taste better and save you money. It may take a bit of initial organization, but eating this way can be almost as quick as heating up a ready-made meal and often far more enjoyable. It just means centering your diet on vitamin-rich fresh produce, protein foods such as lean meat, low-fat dairy, fish and eggs, combined with whole-grain cereals and legumes to supply all the nutrients your body requires.

By handling foods in their whole, original form, you can ensure that each ingredient you use is good quality. For instance, if you cook a fresh fish fillet, or a whole fish, its freshness will be more obvious from its appearance and smell. If you buy prebattered or bread-crumbed fish, it is far more difficult to judge. When you crack an egg for yourself, you can check that it is really fresh: the yolk will stand up to attention, supported by a thick, cloudy, jelly-like white. It looks quite different from an old egg, which will be runny, with a tendency for the yolk to break into the white. An old egg will also float when placed in water, while a fresh egg will sink.

KNOW WHAT YOU'RE EATING

Preparing most of your own meals puts you in charge of their content, giving you every incentive to eat better. If you rely on takeout and fast food, it's much easier to eat badly.

This is why people who eat a lot of takeout and restaurant food often find it hard to control their weight. Although a few convenience-food brands aimed at healthy eaters do make a point of emphasizing that they are full of fruits and vegetables, the vast majority of convenience foods are top-heavy with fat, salt, and carbohydrates. Takeout food is often laden with fat, with few or no vegetables.

If you eat food that's not homemade only once in a while, this is not so important, but if such food forms the backbone of your diet, there can—and most likely will—be negative consequences for your health.

COOKING TO SAVE MONEY AND TIME

If you are not in the habit of cooking regularly, getting geared up to do so can seem daunting. Assembling the ingredients you need for a recipe might, at first, seem off-puttingly expensive, especially in a single or two-person household. If your kitchen is not stocked up with the basics, it might cost, for instance, around $40—much more than the price of a takeout meal—just to buy what you need to cook a meal for two.

Don't be put off. As you build up your pantry, you'll soon find that you're spending much less, and getting significantly better value, than you would if buying convenience food. There is no need to buy everything at once. To minimize cost and effort, do it in stages, perhaps buying a new spice as you try out a new recipe. With your new collection of standby food essentials, and a few tried-and-tested recipes under your belt, you will always be able to put together healthy, affordable, cooked meals.

PANTRY STANDBYS

Here are some suggestions and where to store them; the choice of course, is up to you.

IN THE FRIDGE
- Parmesan cheese, cheddar cheese, feta
- Low-fat natural yogurt (check "Use By" dates)
- A selection of mustards
- Garlic or chili pastes

IN THE FREEZER
- Frozen vegetables (peas and leaf spinach; also green beans, corn, broad beans, edamame beans)
- Salmon, chicken breasts, lean ground meat, small packs of shrimp (individual portions are best as they can be quickly defrosted)
- Homemade stock
- Chilies and herbs (coriander, basil, mint)
- Frozen yogurt and sorbets
- Ready-to-unroll pastry

- Whole-grain pita breads and tortilla wraps
- Frozen berry mixes (often great value compared to fresh, and you can just use the amount you need)

IN THE CUPBOARD

- Canned tuna, sardines, salmon
- Canned corn, plum tomatoes, assortment of beans, tomato purée
- Artichokes, anchovies, sun-dried tomatoes (in oil)
- Capers, pickles
- White wine, red wine, balsamic vinegars
- Tabasco, Worcestershire sauce
- Olive oil, extra virgin olive oil, canola oil
- Sesame oil, soy sauce, Chinese rice wine, Chinese vinegar
- Dried herbs and spices, black pepper
- Flour (whole grain, plain, and self-rising), cornmeal
- Assorted dried pasta (spaghetti, lasagna sheets, penne), couscous
- Egg and rice noodles
- Brown and white rice, oats
- Lentils, split peas, dried beans
- Nuts and seeds (walnuts, almonds, brazils, poppy seeds, pine nuts, sesame seeds)
- Tahini paste
- Rice cakes, whole-grain crackers
- Honey
- Reduced-fat coconut milk or a block of creamed coconut

- Onions, garlic, potatoes

- Canned fruit in their own juice

- Dried fruit (raisins, apricots, apple)

BEYOND THE BASICS

Supplement your pantry items with fresher, more perishable foods (fruits, vegetables, meat, and fish) either weekly or when you need them. Buy a pot of fresh coriander to enliven a simple soup made from your store of legumes, tomatoes, onions, and garlic—and launch your home herb collection. Supplementing pantry staples such as rice and chicken stock with just two additional items—some fresh Parmesan and an onion, for example—you can make a tasty and nutritious risotto.

As you explore new recipes and buy new ingredients, your pantry will soon grow to reflect your personal tastes and eating habits. Having basics on hand, plus more interesting items such as specialty oils, exotic seasonings, and spices, will expand your capacity to provide instant and interesting healthy meals.

Home cooking also saves money by enabling you to take full advantage of foods in season. Newly ripe fruit and vegetables, especially if locally produced, can be far cheaper than out-of-season imports. At a farmers' or produce market, the seasons are visible in the food on display, with new arrivals flagged. What's available will remind you, for instance, that April to June is the time to buy fresh asparagus, or that November is when the clementine season comes into full swing.

Processed food is much the same year-round. If you always head for the processed food shelves, seasonal harvests and the ripe nutrients that they bring will pass you by.

EASY DISHES TO MAKE QUICKLY FROM SCRATCH

Using some of your pantry basics—plus a few fresh ones—you can make many quick, healthy meals. Look at the Eatwell Plate on page 96 to ensure that you get the right balance of nutrients. Here are some ideas:

- Eggs: boiled, poached, scrambled, or as an omelet. For a Spanish-type omelet on a potato base, add mushrooms, vegetables, ham, and cheese.

- Chopped tomatoes with capers, anchovies, and fresh herbs, served with some good-quality ham or cooked chicken on warm pasta or bruschetta.

- Baked or microwaved potatoes in their skins, with protein fillings such as tuna, cheese, or ground beef, served with a salad or other vegetables.

- Smoked fish—such as haddock—baked, grilled, or poached, and served with a poached egg, spinach, and potatoes, or crusty whole-grain bread.

Tips to get the best out of good food

You want your cooking to be as delicious and healthy as possible. Here are a few ideas to help retain flavor and nutrients:

- To reduce the loss of water-soluble vitamins, steam vegetables instead of boil them; bake or roast vegetables such as carrots, parsnips, onions, peppers, or squash; or quickly stir-fry chopped vegetables using a splash of liquid and minimal oil.

- Bake fish in a foil envelope; or microwave or steam to ensure it retains its moistness, natural flavor, and nutrients.

- Roast or grill meat and poultry, and where possible, use the nutritious cooking juices in a gravy or sauce. An inexpensive gravy separator jug, with a spout rising from the bottom, can be a great help to skim the fat off the juice from a roast.

- To minimize the fat in roasted meat, especially for fattier cuts such as lamb or pork shoulder, cook the meat on a rack above the roasting pan to allow the fat to drain out.

- Grilled meat or fish, served with two or three quickly cooked vegetables, pepper, and any herbs you have on hand.

- Stir-fried vegetables (you can buy them frozen), with noodles, shrimp, chicken, or meat, plus herbs and spices. There are dozens of variations.

START-THEN-LEAVE-ALONE DISHES

Slow-cooked, one-pot casserole and stew dishes are simplicity itself. They can take several hours to cook, but are quick to prepare so don't occupy much of your time. To make a simple stew, for example, you need only to brown the meat (already trimmed and cut up by the butcher) with chopped onion; add herbs and aromatics, water, wine (if you have it), or other liquid such as chopped canned tomatoes; then cover and put it in the oven to cook. Give it a stir from time to time, and add other vegetables, such as carrots or mushrooms, as cooking progresses so they don't overcook, then finally add pepper and herbs to taste toward the end of cooking. To make life really simple, put some potatoes into or alongside the casserole.

Slow-cooked dishes of this type allow you to use more economical, lean cuts of meat, such as stewing steak, shin of beef, neck of lamb, or lean diced pork, which many find have more flavor than expensive prime cuts. Vegetarian one-pot meals—such as Boston baked beans, or a spicy chickpea and vegetable stew—are equally low effort, producing cheap and delicious food that is particularly welcome on a cold winter's day.

TIME-EFFECTIVE COOKING

Putting home-cooked meals at the heart of your diet doesn't mean you must cook from scratch every day. With a bit of forethought and organization, one stint of cooking can feed you and your family up to three times. A big Sunday roast is an obvious candidate; leftovers are easily revamped into different meals.

Periodically, set aside a morning or afternoon, or a couple of hours twice a week, to generate food that will serve more than one meal, then chill or freeze the rest. If you're making shepherd's pie, for example, cook double the ingredients and freeze half—either with its mashed potato topping, or add that next time.

Concentrated bursts of cooking can save a huge amount of time and effort later. If you can organize yourself in this way, and remember to take things out of the freezer when required, with minimal reheating you will always have something nice and homemade to eat. Leftovers can always be served up again in the same form as first time, or tweaked to make a different meal.

Here are a few ideas for using one basic dish to produce further meals—with practice, you'll discover many more.

- **Beyond the Sunday roast**—A traditional roast dinner can generate many further possibilities. At its simplest, leftover roast meat can be used for weekday lunches in sandwiches or salads, reducing the amount of salty, processed meat you eat. Or a small amount of chicken can go a long way in a risotto. Once the carcass has been picked clean, it can be simmered with vegetables and aromatics to make stock for soup or to use as a base in another casserole. If you have leftover lamb, you can make a tasty curry, or use leftover beef, plus a can of tomatoes and red kidney beans, to make a quick chili con carne. Or try meat patties: blitz the meat in a food processor, dip in egg and breadcrumbs, then brush with a little olive oil and fry on a griddle.

- **Reinventing leftovers**—Leftover risotto, for example, dressed with a little lemon juice or balsamic vinegar, extra salad vegetables, or cooked meat for more protein, makes a tasty packed lunch.

- **Soups and stews**—Similarly, any chunky vegetable soup can be eaten over one or two days, or on the second day you could turn it into a stew. Add a grain, such as pearl barley or spelt, some fresh green leaves (spinach or finely shredded cabbage), and/or fresh herbs, then drizzle it with olive oil and serve it with grated Parmesan cheese as a vegetable stew. Include cooked meat to make it more substantial or soybeans as a vegetarian option.

- **Same main item, different presentation**—Make a big stew and serve it up with mashed potatoes and cabbage, then freeze the leftover stew to be brought out later and topped with pastry to make a pie. Meanwhile, any leftover potato and cabbage can be added to a soup or mashed together and used as a topping for a fish or meat pie.

- **Different dishes from the same ingredients**—Using ground meat plus a few of your pantry basics, you could try the following:

  1. Mix together ground meat, chopped onions, parsley, egg yolks, any fresh herbs you fancy, plus spices and pepper. Take one half of the mixture and form it into patties or burgers that you grill or fry, and serve with hot vegetables or salad in a wholegrain bun, with pickles on the side. With the rest of the mixture, make meatballs and cook them gently in a bubbling tomato sauce made with lightly sautéed onion and garlic, olive oil and canned tomatoes. Chill or freeze the meatballs in tomato sauce and serve them with pasta on another day.

  2. Or use the ground meat to make a Bolognese-style sauce. Serve half with spaghetti for dinner and put the other half into a lasagna to serve with a fresh green salad the next day. Or flavor half the sauce with a touch of cinnamon, then roast eggplant halves (30 minutes in a hot oven). Fill them with the meat mixture and bake (covered) for 10 minutes, until the eggplant is melting and the filling is bubbling hot.

BREAKFAST REVIEW

When you get up in the morning, it may be ten or twelve hours since you last ate or drank. Your blood sugar will be at a fasting level. Without sustenance, your body has to call on its energy reserves, and you may feel tired, despite your sleep, and possibly unwell. Breakfast provides an effective supply of dietary glucose to fuel the start of your day.

TOP OFF YOUR TANK

Liquid is the first requirement. You lose moisture every time you exhale—breathe on a mirror to see the effect. Moisture escapes through your skin as well. Overnight, this adds up to about a mugful. The body has also been making urine as it deals with consumption from the previous evening. To process and excrete a dinner with a high salt content, especially if accompanied by alcohol and followed by caffeine, requires another mug or two of water from the body. To replace all this:

- Start with a glass of water, before moving on to your preferred morning drink, such as tea or coffee, juice or milk.

- Most adults need to drink at least 1.2 liters (40 ounces) of liquid over the course of the day; you should drink around a third of that within an hour of getting up.

- Drink something you like. Research suggests that, when asked to drink more water and cut down on beverages and soft drinks, people drank less fluid altogether. But limit caffeine drinks to no more than five a day.

NO EXCUSE NOT TO EAT

Most health experts recommend a breakfast that gives you at least 300 calories and some say much more. Not everyone feels hungry first thing in the morning and many of us are in a rush. But lack of time is no reason to skip breakfast. It takes just a few minutes to eat a bowl of cereal, down a yogurt drink, or munch a slice of whole-grain toast and peanut butter . . . and you really don't need to feel hungry to do so.

WHAT BREAKFAST SHOULD SUPPLY

A bigger breakfast will sustain you for longer. Try to think of it on a plate, with representatives from your "food friends": complex carbohydrates, protein, dairy foods, fats, and fruits or vegetables. Aim for a combination of these to supply the energy and range of nutrients you need to keep going through the morning.

You might think that by eating little or no breakfast, you're saving calories for the day. That's not how hunger works. Breakfast is the meal that most successfully regulates the hunger-stimulating hormone ghrelin, keeping levels low, which reduces hunger and food cravings throughout the day. A number of studies have found that eating a balanced breakfast is important for weight control, as well as general well-being.

BREAKFAST CEREALS— WHAT DO THEY OFFER?

People in as many as 140 countries now start their day with breakfast cereals. Most of us choose packaged cereals for convenience. They can be a perfectly healthy option, too. Just make sure you opt for whole-grain, low-sugar, and low-salt products, and avoid those that are heavily processed.

COMPLEX OAT CEREALS

These may take a little longer to prepare and eat but many oat-based cereals provide better, longer-lasting sustenance. If the ingredient list is short and simple, you can see at a glance exactly what you are getting.

- **Muesli and granola**—Raw rolled oats mixed with nuts, seeds, and dried fruits supply a rich variety of nutrients, especially when combined with the protein and calcium of milk or yogurt. Oats are slow to digest, and with the protein and fiber of nuts, provide a lasting feeling of fullness, plus the beta glucan in oats helps keep blood-cholesterol levels low. But check the nutrition labels, especially of sweetened and toasted granola varieties, as these products can be high in fat and calories. Add berries and fruits—frozen berries are a nutritious alternative when fresh are out of season.

- **Oatmeal**—Unrefined whole rolled or steel-cut oats are a rich source of the soluble fiber beta glucan, which removes cholesterol from the intestine, and also supplies vitamin E, which scavenges and neutralizes damaging free radicals. Buy unrefined oats in preference to instant oats, which are more processed and have a higher GI (glycemic index), making them less filling.

  Preparing oatmeal with milk improves the protein quality of the oats, as well as adding calcium. Seasonal berries and fruits add vitamins and phytochemicals, and further enhance the fiber content. Manuka honey, believed to have antibiotic qualities, adds natural sweetness. Walnuts crumbled on top add vitamin E, essential fatty acids, and a satisfying crunch.

BREADS AND BUNS

Many of us enjoy toast at breakfast. It's warm, smells good as it cooks, and holds toppings well. So what type of bread should you toast? Eating whole grains may help prevent heart disease, but store-bought whole-grain or seeded breads are not necessarily the healthiest choice.

- Whole-grain wheat bread with lots of seeds supplies protein with a rich mix of fiber, essential fatty acids, and vitamins A, D, and E. However, many breads and rolls—including some of the best-looking seeded varieties—also contain much more salt than you would add to a home-baked loaf.

- White bread lacks the fiber of whole grains, but is still nutritious. Bread flour is fortified with calcium, iron, and B vitamins thiamin and niacin to replace those lost in the milling process. As with whole-grain and wheat bread, salt levels vary.

So, which is best? The ingredients label of a store-bought loaf—white or brown—is your best guide. If the bread contains more than 1 gram of salt per 100 grams, some health experts say it's too high.

WHAT TO SPREAD ON BREAD

Many people still consume unhealthy amounts of saturated fat each day, which can contribute to heart disease. Butter is one particular source, so this may be where you should cut back, if necessary.

Health experts suggest that fats should supply no more than about a third of our total daily calories, and that saturated fat should make up, at most, a third of total fat. That's a suggested maximum of less than 2 ounces (4 tablespoons) of butter a day, with no saturated fats from any other sources, such as meat. Butter is the gold standard for taste and "melt in the mouth" sensation, but if you tend to eat too much saturated fat, consider instead using olive and sunflower oil–based spreads, light, fat-reduced spreads, or cholesterol-lowering spreads.

Additional spreads are often a question of individual taste; some have a few nutritional benefits, but most have drawbacks, as well:

- **Jam** brings sugar but only a trace of vitamins—look for high-fruit-content varieties. Some reduced-sugar jams use concentrated grape juice to add sweetness.

- **Honey** has more fructose than regular jam, which gives it an intensely sweet taste. You need only a little, especially if it is a pure blossom honey, which has a stronger flavor.

- **Peanut butter** raises the protein quality and quantity when added to bread, producing a highly nutritious and satiating food. Look for low-salt and low-sugar varieties.

- **Hazelnut-chocolate spread,** like peanut butter, increases protein quality, but it also adds sugar and fat. It's best used sparingly.

THE BIG BREAKFAST— WHAT TO EMBRACE AND WHAT TO AVOID

Eggs are a good choice. They are highly nutritious and relatively cheap. An egg provides around 6.5 grams of protein—13 percent of the adult daily requirement. Eggs are a good source of the vitamin D we need—especially in winter, when there's little sunshine. They contain the B vitamins riboflavin, biotin, folate, and also B_{12}, which can be lacking in vegetarian diets since their best source is animals. Eggs also supply iodine, vitamin A, zinc, phosphorus, iron, selenium, and some omega-3 fats.

With about 280 milligrams of cholesterol per egg, there has been concern that eggs raise cholesterol levels in blood, but various scientific studies are challenging this. One twelve-week study found that people on a low-calorie diet who ate two eggs a day not only lost weight, but also reduced their cholesterol levels. For most healthy people, the dietary intake of cholesterol, especially from low-fat foods such as eggs, has little impact on blood cholesterol levels.

Eggs are particularly good at increasing satiety—feelings of fullness—and decreasing hunger. One or two eggs served with a piece of whole-grain toast makes an excellent breakfast, but don't add extra salt.

Boiling or poaching eggs adds no extra calories (except for those in a drop of oil, if you are using a poaching pan). Frying does increase the calorie count, so it's best to use a nonstick frying pan and a little olive oil. For scrambled eggs, mix one or two eggs with a drop of milk, and cook with a little oil in a nonstick pan, then serve on whole-grain toast.

OTHER OPTIONS

- **Avoid hash browns.** Imagine soaking a small sponge in fat, then frying it. Hash browns are like starchy sponges full of fat—best avoided.

- **Limit breakfast meats,** sausages, and bacon. The World Cancer Research Fund reports a link between eating processed meat and increased risk of bowel cancer. They recommend that meats that have been smoked, cured, or have added preservatives (such as ham, bacon, and some sausages) should be restricted in the diet. A healthier breakfast choice is to add a little smoked salmon to scrambled eggs.

- **Orange juice** makes the most of the iron in eggs. The body's absorption of iron is enhanced when eggs are eaten with a source of vitamin C, which is one reason why fresh orange juice is a good choice at breakfast.

- **Tea** isn't a good choice with eggs. The tannin in strong black tea binds to the iron in eggs and impedes its absorption into the body.

- **Yogurt** is made by heating and cooling milk, then adding a bacteria culture that ferments the lactose into lactic acid. As a result of the slightly denatured protein, the reduced amount of lactose, and the presence of a bacteria culture, many people find yogurt easier to digest than milk. Some yogurts come in semiliquid form for pouring over cereal or fruit.

BREAKFAST BEVERAGES

COFFEE

Over the years, the reputation of coffee has swung from good to bad and back again. Recent favorable studies suggest that the benefits of consuming up to 5 cups a day may be:

- A lower risk of developing Parkinson's disease and Alzheimer's disease.

- Better bowel mobility, which may help prevent constipation.

- Better cognitive performance, especially in later life.

It seems that drinking some coffee is good for most of us. But not all: pregnant women are advised to avoid it as caffeine passes through the placenta and lingers in the developing baby ten times longer than in an adult.

Many people also get "coffee jitters" if they drink more than a few cups of strong coffee. The caffeine can produce sleep problems if consumed later in the day.

The espresso brewing method produces the best-quality coffee (with not too much caffeine), lots of taste, and the highest yield of antioxidants. French-press coffee comes second for quality, with more caffeine. The hotter the water and the longer the beans or grinds are immersed, the more caffeine is available.

TEA

Black tea offers some caffeine to help wake us up and also contains disease-fighting molecules called catechins, although levels are higher in green teas. Two other phytochemicals are present in trace amounts—theobromine and theophylline, which are used medicinally to treat asthma and other respiratory diseases. Many studies have examined the possible role of tea in reducing rates of cancer, but the results have been inconclusive.

MILK AND YOGURT DRINKS

Dairy products contribute important nutrients to the breakfast meal. A cup of milk, alone or in a bowl of cereal, supplies around 16 percent of daily protein needs and about 40 percent of daily calcium needs, plus riboflavin, pantothenic acid, vitamin B_{12}, phosphorus, and iodine.

Young children should have whole milk, especially if they are very active. Low-fat or skim milk is a better option for adults who have to be more careful with the calorie and fat content of their diets. Other available milks and milk products include:

- **Soy milk**—The fresh chilled varieties have a pleasant taste and come sweetened or unsweetened. The contents are about

5 percent soybeans, with added calcium and vitamins. A cup of soy milk contains around 6 grams of protein. Some people with an intolerance to the natural sugar in cow's milk (lactose) find soy milk a useful alternative.

- **Yogurt-type drinks**—These are sold as a daily nutrient boost in small, individual bottles. Some contain acidophilus strains of bacteria to increase the population of friendly bacteria in the gut, and some contain plant sterols with cholesterol-lowering properties.

JUICES—THE FRESHER THE BETTER

Juices make a refreshing start to the day and are a good source of vitamins, minerals, and phytochemicals; one serving counts as one of your recommended five-a-day fruits and vegetables. However, most juices contain more than 100 calories per 8½-ounce glass, so keep the glass small or dilute the juice with some water.

BREAKFAST ON THE RUN

A quick breakfast can still be nutritious. Always have a drink, then take breakfast food with you. Here are a few portable suggestions:

- Six walnuts or almonds, or four Brazil nuts.

- A few dried prunes or apricots.

- Yogurt—probiotic or soy, if preferred.

- Small peanut butter sandwich on whole-grain bread.

- Smoothie made with fresh fruit and yogurt.

- Pita filled with ricotta and berries.

- Piece of fruit, plus a yogurt drink.

Chapter 20

HEALTHY SNACKS

It's natural to feel hungry between meals, which may be five hours or more apart. A medium-size meal takes one to two hours to pass through the stomach, before continuing along the small intestine. Blood glucose rises soon after eating but within a few hours falls back to its normal level, and the brain begins to signal hunger. The best type of snack plugs the gap so we reach our next meal ready for food but not ravenous.

We may dismiss feelings of hunger when distracted by an absorbing activity, but then the body has to draw on other energy reserves to supply glucose to our brains and tissues, which can make us feel tired. If the gap between meals is too great, our brains know we need energy, and hunger can become so intense that we eat too much at the next meal. Healthy snacks between meals can help keep hunger under control.

WHO WANTS A SNACK?

A typical daily snacking schedule might be breakfast/SNACK/ lunch/SNACK/dinner. The urge to snack will hit at different times, depending on individual patterns of activity or stages in life.

- **Early risers**—Anyone who eats breakfast around 7 a.m., especially those who do physical work, will need a substantial snack midmorning.

Four tips for sensible snacking

A snack is satisfying when it produces feelings of satiety and passes slowly through the digestive system. Top nutritionists recommend:

- Protein from foods such as cheese, eggs, hummus, or peanut butter.

- Fat, preferably "good" fats, such as those in nuts or avocados.

- Complex carbs from snacks such as oatcakes or whole-grain foods.

- A twenty-minute pause after snacking so your brain can register the effect.

- **Late diners**—If lunch is around 1 p.m., anyone who will eat dinner later than 7 p.m. may need something late afternoon to avoid the hunger-driven temptation to pick at anything available.

- **The young**—Children don't eat large meals and need healthy snacks throughout the day to maintain their high-energy and nutrient levels.

- **Adolescents**—Even though teenagers might eat lots at mealtimes, the growing body makes high demands on energy and nutrients, so regular, healthy snacks are essential.

- **The very active**—Fit, sporty adults who exercise frequently need to boost energy and nutrient intake between meals.

- **The elderly**—By contrast, retired people may eat breakfast later, followed by smaller but more frequent meals and an earlier dinner. Unless they are very active during the day, an appropriate snack could be as light as a nutritious drink or piece of fruit.

WHAT MAKES A GOOD SNACK?

What you choose to snack on matters. It not only affects your appetite and what you eat at mealtimes, but can also influence how effectively you function throughout the day. A good snack will do three things:

- Boost your daily nutrient intake

- Plug a hunger gap

- Give you a feeling of well-being

A stick of celery might help with the first, but it will likely leave you unsatisfied and won't get you through to the next meal. Treats may fail on all three counts, as any satisfaction may be disappointingly short lived. Sugary treats are also digested very quickly, so you're soon feeling hungry again. Then you eat more, setting a dangerous precedent.

Here are some examples of snacks that meet all three "good snack" conditions—they are nutritionally sound, help fill a gap, and are delicious enough to be satisfying, too. First is a category that you might not suspect could be good for you.

BAKED GOODS

These get a bad press, but scones and English muffins are low in fat, and the wheat flour is a source of protein, calcium, and B vitamins. Since processed versions usually contain too much salt, go for home-baked, and use whole-grain flour. The basic ingredients—milk, flour, and butter—supply essential nutrients, and you control the fat, sugar, and salt content:

- Homemade scones can be sweet or savory: raisin, cheese and chive, date, or pumpkin. They are best eaten the day they are made, but they freeze well, too.

- Banana bread and raisin and bran muffins are further

examples of healthy homemade snacks. The loaves can be sliced and frozen in batches; muffins also freeze well.

FRUITS

A couple of pieces a day adds the sweetness we often crave and helps us achieve our daily requirements for vitamin C, folic acid, and fiber, plus important phytochemicals. Where possible, buy fruit in season; it tastes better and has more nutrients. Always wash fruit to remove dirt and pesticide traces. Apples, pears, and bananas are good staples. Easy-peel tangerines are practical and packed with vitamin C. In winter, oranges are at their best: sweet and delicious and well worth the effort of peeling. Red grapes, berries, and cherries pack a terrific antioxidant boost. Orange- and red-colored exotic fruits—such as papaya, mango, and cantaloupe—are rich in carotenoid phytochemicals that aid good eye function.

LIQUID SNACKS

There is a tasty variety of smoothies and yogurt drinks available, but always check the ingredients, as some are sweetened and contain too much sugar and unnecessary additives. You should also keep these points in mind:

- **Smoothies** that contain the whole fruit pulp rather than just the juice have plenty of fiber. A daily whole-fruit smoothie can count as one of your recommended five-a-day fruit and veggie portions.

- **Yogurt drinks** can be pure yogurt or a mixture of yogurt with juice. They tend to be easily digested, provide valuable calcium and phosphorus, and have a high protein content that helps us feel full. But again, check labels to avoid additives and flavorings.

- **Probiotic yogurt drinks** have strains of acidophilus bacteria added to help maintain a healthy population of bacteria in the intestine. Intestinal bacteria provide us with certain essential fatty acids and two-thirds of our daily intake of vitamin K.

- **Milky drinks,** such as lattes and cappuccinos, can feel satisfying even when made with low-fat milk. But beware the fashionable hijacking of this healthy snack through the addition of unnecessary sugar, flavored syrup, or cream.

RAW NUTS

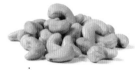

Nuts are highly nutritious, so just a few are sufficient for a healthy snack. A handful of mixed dried fruits and nuts, well wrapped and carried in a lunch box or handbag, is an excellent portable snack. Nuts contain

Hearty snacks

If you get home late in the afternoon and go out again to play a sport or take part in an activity that will delay your evening meal, you will need a substantial snack to keep you going for a few hours. Here are some suggestions:

- Pita bread toasted and filled with hummus, plus grated carrot or tomato.

- Half a small ciabatta, toasted and spread with pesto, avocado, and tomato.

- Slice of whole-grain toast, spread with peanut butter or low-fat cheese.

- Two rice cakes with ricotta or cottage cheese.

- Hummus with sticks of carrot, celery, or cucumber, or raw cauliflower florets.

- Yogurt drink with a banana is ideal before playing a sport— easily digested carbohydrates, protein, plus a calcium and potassium boost.

- Half an avocado with a little olive oil, balsamic vinegar, and black pepper.

essential unsaturated "good" fats, plus phytosterols that inhibit the absorption of "bad" LDL cholesterol. A number of studies suggest that they help heart health.

- **Brazil and cashew nuts** are particularly rich in selenium, which is essential for healthy thyroid function.

- **Pistachios** are the nuts that are lowest in fat and highest in protein.

- **Nut spreads**—such as peanut and almond butter—make a great snack on a rice cake or small piece of whole-grain or rye bread.

AVOID THE SNACKING DANGER ZONES

With tempting snacks all too readily available, it's easy to succumb despite our best intentions. Here are a few of the most common snack traps and simple ways to arm yourself against them or, at least, mitigate their effects.

DANGER ZONE ONE: PEER-PRESSURE SNACKING

Sharing food and drink with friends and family at home or work is one of life's most pleasurable rituals. Yet, when unhealthy, highly tempting foods are seemingly ubiquitous it can have an unwelcome impact on health. In one research study, 64 percent of office employees felt that coworkers brought too many cakes and treats into the office; 24 percent said they couldn't resist them; and 14 percent felt pressured to join in eating them. It feels rude to refuse, so if everyone is sharing a celebration cake or cookies, you join in, even though you might be trying to watch your weight and know that this is not the healthiest choice. Here are some tips to buck the trend for treats without causing a riot:

- **Timetable the treats**—While an everyday cookie or cake habit is unwise, a complete absence of food treats at work seems unfriendly and unnecessary. As a compromise, try to encourage healthy snacks as the norm, with treats being kept, say, for Friday afternoons or, better still, for more special occasions.

- **Turn peer pressure into peer support**—People are more successful at making changes to poor eating habits when they seek help from friends and family. Getting a few key allies to support you in a quest to include healthier foods is likely to be more successful than tackling the issue alone.

- **Make the first move**—At work or at home, be the first to introduce a selection of healthy snacks to nibble on, such as: in-season strawberries, grapes, peaches, figs or apricots, pistachios or other nuts, small packets of dried fruit, or rice cakes.

Once a daily habit of healthy snacks is established, a treat will be appreciated all the more. Encourage homemade cakes and muffins, as they will probably contain healthier ingredients. More indulgent offerings, too, are perfectly acceptable—once in a while and in small portions.

DANGER ZONE TWO: SNACKS WITH ALCOHOL

Most of us know we should eat something when we're drinking alcohol. The problem is that healthy snacks are seldom available in bars. Most bar snacks are salty—a deliberate ploy designed to make us drink more. If salted chips and nuts are the only options, limit the portion size by sharing, and don't make them a habit. If you are serving drinks at home, or whenever the place or situation allows:

SWAP THE BAD GUYS . . .

- Salted roasted peanuts

- Potato chips

- Root vegetable chips: healthy perception but similar calorie, fat, and salt content

- Corn chips with salsa

. . . FOR THE GOOD GUYS

- **Raw peanuts**—high in protein, magnesium, and zinc, more B vitamins and iron, no salt and less fat than salted, roasted versions.

- **Nuts in shells, such as pistachios and raw peanuts**—slower to eat (since you have to shell them) and a good source of essential fatty acids. In one study, when two groups were given shelled or unshelled nuts to eat, those who had to shell the nuts ate 50 percent fewer but felt equally satisfied. The pile of empty shells also gives a visual cue of the quantity consumed.

- **Hummus with veggie sticks**—low in calories and all goodness—protein and fiber from the chickpeas, blended with olive oil.

- **Edamame beans (soft young soybeans)**—high in protein and fiber, and a good source of thiamin, folate, and iron. They are best bought frozen, then briefly blanched. Like nuts, these beans need to be shelled from their pods, so are quite fun to eat.

GOOD NEWS AND BAD NEWS

- Olives are low calorie and rich in good monounsaturated fat, but most are very salty: 2 or 3 olives contain around 13 percent of the maximum daily limit.

- Pretzels are low in calories but are almost pure carbohydrate with few useful nutrients. And like most salted snack foods, they have too much salt.

- Popcorn is low in calories and high in fiber but has a high glycemic index (GI), so it is quickly digested and not a suitable snack for diabetics on its own.

DANGER ZONE THREE: JUST GOT HOME AND STARVING

A particular snacking danger zone occurs when we are hungry enough to eat a full meal but have to wait. One of the most common times for this is when we arrive home from a day at school or work. Dinner may still be a few hours away, so raiding the fridge is common practice—and the hungrier we are, the less careful we are about what we eat. We want instant gratification, so healthy snacks need to be available fast, or the temptation to pig out on cookies, salty crackers, or chocolate can be too hard to resist. Here are some tips to help you avoid this danger zone:

- **Pack a snack.** If you carry a healthy snack to eat shortly before leaving work, or even on the way home, you will avoid arriving home feeling ravenous. A cup of tea or piece of fruit will be enough.

- **Stock up on healthy snacks.** Make sure the fridge always contains easy snacks such as yogurt drinks, hummus and carrots, or ricotta cheese to spread on rice cakes. Always have fresh fruit available.

- **Plan what you will eat.** If you get home without any idea of what you are going to snack on and start browsing the cupboards for anything edible, it is all too easy to eat too much of the wrong stuff. It is better to know in advance what the snack is going to be. Children and young people especially benefit from being told what to go for. If they know, for example, to help themselves to a post-school snack of a bowl of cereal, a yogurt drink, or a piece of whole-grain toast with peanut butter, this removes a large part of the anxiety caused by feeling hungry. They can be quickly satisfied and move on to other activities.

- **Don't bring the bad guys into the house.** If chips and cookies are in the house, they're going to get eaten and ruin even the best intentions of snacking well. High-fat, salty, and sugary foods can be irresistible when arriving home hungry. Think of them as treat foods that are bought in small quantities for specific occasions, not as a regular feature in your diet.

- **Don't mistake thirst for hunger.** When we arrive home from a day out anywhere, it's likely that we're thirsty, and to avoid fatigue we need to rehydrate rather than eat. Our brains can often confuse these two needs. A glass of water is perfect, perhaps followed by a smoothie or yogurt drink. Tea is great to help de-stress; a cup of coffee is also fine, as long as it is large enough to quench thirst.

- **Beware of opportunist snacking.** As many moms know, children's snack-time leftovers can be a dangerous temptation. When the kids leave tasty morsels on the plate, it is easy to justify polishing them off as "avoiding waste." Don't eat for the sake of it, or feel you have to eat up leftovers. Plan to have a small, snack-size share or have a healthy alternative on hand.

DANGER ZONE FOUR: "NEED A LIFT" NIBBLES

These moments can occur when we aren't even hungry—the urge to eat is a "substitute" desire. It could stem from feeling a bit unsettled, or perhaps bored, or having to wait for something or someone. A snack fills the gap, and a treat affords a bit of short-lived pleasure. But when "need a lift" nibbles become too regular, they can become an unhealthy habit. Avoid the danger by training yourself to switch to an alternative. Here are some tips:

- **Drink something not associated with snacking.** Try chilled, carbonated water, a calming peppermint tea, or an infusion of hot water with a slice of fresh ginger and lemon.

- **Perform a substitute mood-raising activity.** Get some exercise: do ten squats, or lie on the carpet and do ten tummy crunches. Alternatively, phone a friend, switch on the radio, or do a bit of personal pampering, such as moisturizing your hands.

- **Suck a mint or chew gum.** The action of sucking has a calming sensation that is hardwired into the brain from the earliest moments of infancy. When you are an adult, it can still bring relief from tension. A sweet mint flavor can also reduce cravings for other foods.

- **Ban unhealthy treats from the house.** If you do this, you won't be presented with irresistible temptation. If you must eat, go for something chewy, such as dried mango or apricot.

- **Postpone the nibble.** Decide what you're going to nibble on, but put off actually doing it for fifteen minutes. There is a good chance that the desire will subside, especially if you get effectively distracted by some activity.

DANGER ZONE FIVE: NIGHTTIME MUNCHIES

Feeling hungry at night can happen when:

- Dinner is eaten very early.

- The evening meal wasn't substantial enough.

- You've been very active and need an energy boost.

- You have digestive problems and can only eat small portions.

Nighttime snacking doesn't have to be a danger zone, but can be if the nibbles are unhealthily high in fat, sugar, or salt. When you eat early and then relax at home in front of the

Reader's Digest Quintessential Guide

television, you're probably aware that TV food commercials or even cooking shows are a potential snack trigger. Don't succumb to an urge that is not a need—but if you do succumb, make sure that you eat fruit or something equally healthy rather than chips, cookies, or cake. Dark chocolate can be a satisfying snack because its bitterness, countered with just enough sweetness, makes it pleasant but not so sweet that you want to eat the whole bar. Two squares of dark chocolate with a low-fat cappuccino tastes like total indulgence, while being packed with nutrients.

Haphazard daytime eating can lead to "grazing" behavior—snacking on bits and pieces here and there, and never gaining a clear picture of the amount of food actually eaten. A nourishing evening meal—eaten several hours before bedtime to allow digestion but not so early that you become hungry again—is the best way to stay feeling full.

Those with very active lives may need a substantial snack in the late evening, despite an earlier evening meal. Ideal snacks for this time include a bowl of cereal or slice of whole-grain toast, which will supply the energy you need but won't keep you awake.

For others, the classic hot-milk drink is comforting. The protein helps you feel full, while natural sugars add a little sweetness. Homemade cocoa is better than drinking prepared hot chocolate mixes, as you can control the amount of added sugar; ready-prepared chocolate drink powders often have more sugar and less cocoa. Skim or low-fat milk keeps the calorie count down.

Chapter 21

YOUR MIDDAY MEAL

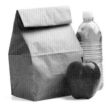

Lunch was once the main meal, but for many working people today it is small or sometimes nonexistent. The tough "lunch is for wimps" office mentality frowns on a midday break, concerned that food wastes time or slows you down. This is wrong and unhealthy for the following reasons:

- A balanced midday meal keeps your metabolism active, supplying the energy to keep you going physically and mentally.

- The right foods help regulate blood-sugar levels so you may avoid the highs and lows that create tiredness and mood swings.

- If you don't eat properly at lunchtime, you're more likely to overeat in the evening, when you are much less likely to be active.

What we eat can determine the degree of post-lunch drowsiness we experience. Refined carbohydrates—such as sugars, white bread, and white rice—produce a rapid rise in blood glucose. As the body releases insulin to control the levels, the liver and muscles extract glucose from the blood and store it, making us feel tired. The release of insulin also prompts the brain to produce the chemicals serotonin and melatonin, which encourage sleep.

By contrast, whole-grain starchy foods have a lower GI, which causes blood-sugar levels to rise more gradually, avoiding energy peaks and troughs. Combining protein foods with complex carbohydrates tends to lower the GI of the meal overall. The result is less postprandial sleepiness.

LUNCH AT HOME

As more of us work from home and others live longer in retirement, we could prepare a delicious hot or cold midday meal. But do we? Many of us simply grab what's there, barely pausing to enjoy it. Why not savor good, healthy food instead? These quick ideas can be whipped up in ten to fifteen minutes.

SPEEDY MEDITERRANEAN-STYLE SALADS

Start with whatever vegetables and lettuce you have on hand, and add leftover cold meat, a hard-boiled egg, or a can of tuna. Finish with a drizzle of olive oil and balsamic vinegar, a sprinkling of sesame seeds, pine nuts or poppy seeds, and serve with a slice of wholegrain bread. For variations, try:

- **Greek**—Chop up tomatoes, feta cheese, cucumber, and red onion. Add in a splash of olive oil and a pinch of dried oregano, and toss before serving.

- **Italian**—Nix the feta from the Greek recipe, but add mozzarella, some fresh basil, and a small amount of crushed garlic.

- **Spanish**—Add a little tasty Manchego cheese and small amounts of chorizo, then top with a few olives.

FRITTATAS AND OMELETS

First, whisk up the eggs and while they are cooking prepare your filling. Serve with crispy salad leaves and a squeeze of lemon juice.

Fill an omelet with chopped ripe avocado and a small handful of grated mature cheddar. Or try crumbled feta and sun-dried tomatoes.

Fry sliced zucchini in a little olive oil and add to a frittata with leftover boiled potatoes and chopped mint.

QUICK SOUP

It takes about ten minutes to steam vegetables (squash, cauliflower, or broccoli) and then whizz them up in a blender with a dash of milk and some fresh herbs. Finish with a spoonful of low-fat crème fraîche or yogurt and a few grinds of black pepper. Try butternut squash with sage, cauliflower with nutmeg, or classic pea with mint. Use pantry ingredients to make a quick fish stew with canned tuna or mackerel plus canned beans and tomatoes, or make a carton of soup healthier and heartier by adding leftover vegetables.

When you have time, cook batches of soup and freeze in individual portions that can be quickly defrosted. You will avoid the salt and processing of canned varieties, and save money.

LUNCH **AT WORK**

Many of us skip lunch on a regular basis. Increasingly, it seems, hectic schedules have pushed lunch to a backseat.

If your workplace provides a fridge and microwave, make use of them. Taking leftovers or homemade soup to reheat at work is an economical way to get a quick, warm, and nourishing meal in the middle of the day. On days when you have nothing suitable, many packaged convenience foods, such

Five rules for safe leftovers

Leftovers can easily be reheated as they are or jazzed up with extra ingredients to make a tasty, nutritious, and easy lunch. Just be sure to follow these rules:

- Cover and cool leftover food as quickly as you can, ideally within ninety minutes. If there's a large amount, separate into smaller portions. Once the food is cool, refrigerate immediately.

- Use refrigerated leftovers within two days. If reheating leftovers, make sure they're piping hot throughout.

- Don't reheat leftovers more than once. Repeatedly warming food increases the amount of time it spends at the ideal temperature for bacterial growth. The longer the food is warm, the more bacteria are able to multiply.

- Cool leftovers completely before freezing. For flavor, they are best eaten within three months, but can safely be kept frozen longer.

- Defrost leftovers completely either in the fridge or in a microwave. Frozen leftovers should be defrosted thoroughly before they are reheated.

as noodles and fresh or dried soups, are designed for people with busy lunchtimes. These may be useful if you're pushed for time, but check the labels carefully to avoid high levels of salt and fat.

LUSCIOUS LUNCH BOXES

While leftovers can make a delicious and economical lunch, they won't always be available. When choosing other lunch-box foods, the challenge is keeping them healthy and interesting. Try out the speedy salads on page 145, but be sure to take the dressing in a separate container so your salad stays crisp. Or you can try out the following:

- Swap ordinary-bread sandwiches for a tasty wrap or lightly toasted and filled pita bread.

- Prepare a mini-buffet of sliced carrots, peppers, cucumbers, and celery to dip in hummus, plus a handful of grapes and nuts for dessert.

- For a quick-and-easy dessert, chop fresh fruit into a container and top with natural yogurt.

- Make a healthy vegetable pâté—mushrooms and lentils work especially well—and eat with breadsticks or slices of carrots and red peppers.

- Roast chicken drumsticks in olive oil, lemon juice, and chopped coriander; make enough for a couple of days and keep refrigerated. Eat with a small salad.

- If you're making dessert the night before that can be eaten cold, make enough for lunch, too—a poached pear, for example, gently cooked in white wine and orange juice flavored with star anise, or a baked apple, cored and filled with raisins, nuts, and honey.

SPICE THEM UP—HEALTHY, DELICIOUS SANDWICHES

Although variety is important at lunchtime, don't ignore the traditional sandwich. Here are some tips on refreshing this lunchtime favorite:

- Try artisan breads—a seeded whole-grain loaf or one with added nuts and cheese, or garlic and olives, or sun-dried tomatoes. The more nutritious your bread, the more nutritious your lunch will be.

- Branch out from the usual mayo and mustard, and use a chutney, relish, or sauce. Try pesto with mozzarella and tomato, or pickled red cabbage with cold roast beef.

- Pack in more flavor by using strong cheeses such as Stilton or Gorgonzola, tasty veggies such as sun-dried tomatoes, and peppery leaves such as arugula and watercress.

Try something different

TRY	WHY?	HOW?
Quinoa— a grain-like seed that looks a bit like couscous	It's a good source of protein and cooks in just ten minutes.	Cook according to packaging instructions and use in salads or in the same way you would rice or pasta. Try it with zucchini, feta, and red onion.
Walnuts and Brazil nuts	Walnuts have been shown to help maintain flexible blood vessels. A handful of Brazils provides your daily selenium requirement, boosting your immune system.	Chop and add to salads or yogurt. Or bake them into a cake, such as a carrot cake.
Sweet potatoes	Orange-fleshed varieties are rich in beta-carotene and are delicious roasted.	Chop into chunks and roast with bell peppers in olive oil. Add a little vinegar and toss with salad leaves.
Flax seeds	A vegetarian source of omega-3 fatty acids.	Take a small container of seeds to sprinkle on top of yogurts and salads just before eating.

- Instead of tuna, try canned crab; it adds immunity-boosting zinc to your diet. Mix it with some chopped spring onions, a small amount of mayonnaise, and a dab of Dijon mustard.

- Go "light" with a carrot and raisin sandwich: peel and grate a carrot; add a few raisins, chopped mint, and black pepper, and bind together with a dollop of hummus.

FEEDING CHILDREN AND TEENS

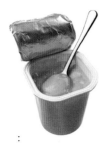

Coming up with healthy lunches for children can be a challenge; their fussy eating habits combined with peer pressure from classmates to choose this or reject that food can make it hard to know what to pack. Most children don't eat healthily enough. One survey of children's lunches showed that more than half contained sweets or chocolate, and nearly half included a salty snack such as chips.

While the quality of food in lunches provided by schools has occasionally been spotlighted, home-packed lunches tend to slip under the quality-control radar. Some schools have adopted special policies aimed at encouraging parents to provide a nutritious packed lunch; these may include a ban on chips, sweets, or chocolate. Even schools without a specific policy often offer guideline recommendations. For a healthy, everyday lunch for your child, try to include:

- At least one portion of fruit and one portion of vegetables.

- Some meat, fish, or other source of nondairy protein, such as lentils, kidney beans, chickpeas, or peanut butter. (Limit processed meats.)

- A starchy food, such as whole-grain bread, pasta, rice, couscous, or potatoes.

- Dairy foods, such as milk, cheese, or yogurt.

- A drink, which could be unsweetened fruit juice, skim or low-fat milk, a yogurt drink, a smoothie, or simply water.

- At least once a week, try to include oily fish, such as salmon.

As children reach their teens and become more independent, they want more control over what and where they eat. Nutritionally, this is an important time. Since their bodies are developing and maturing, you have to give consistent positive messages about food to help keep them on track.

If your teenager's school offers lunches, check the menu and encourage healthy choices. If you have to prepare packed lunches, find time to discuss what food is going into their lunch and why you don't want to include chips, chocolate bars, or sodas. You may find you need to compromise between what you would ideally like them to have, and what they feel is "cool" to eat in front of friends.

Healthy lunch-box swaps for kids (and great for grown-ups, too!)

INSTEAD OF	SWITCH TO
White bread and rolls	Seeded bread, whole-grain mini-rolls, whole-grain pita bread and wraps, oat-based breads and rolls. If your children really don't like "brown" bread, try some of the 50:50 breads available—they are made with 50 percent whole-grain flour, but the taste and texture are more like white bread
Carbonated drinks	Water, milk, diluted fruit juice, smoothies
Cakes	Homemade muffins with added fruit and seeds
Chocolate pudding	Live yogurt with chopped fruit, such as strawberries or grapes
Cookies and candy	Nuts and raisins, dried apple rings, or fruit-and-nut granola bars (but check that sugar content is not too high)
Chips	Plain, air-popped popcorn or, as an occasional treat, unsalted chips
No vegetables	Some vegetable—either in the sandwiches or in separate containers. Try sticks of bright red and orange peppers, raw carrots, cucumbers or crisp celery, with a little pot of hummus as a dip

Many older teens are allowed to eat out of school at lunchtime. It may not be easy, but try to discuss what they are eating in cafés and fast-food restaurants, and encourage them to make healthy choices. Make sure they have snacks containing fruits, vegetables, and whole grains with them for breaks and after school.

EATING OUT AND ABOUT

Whether you're at work or shopping with friends, the options for eating out at lunchtime, particularly in a city center, are more varied than ever. Upmarket sandwich shops and sushi and noodle bars sit alongside the more familiar burger fast-food chains and traditional pubs or cafés. Yet it can be surprisingly difficult to find a lunch that is both healthy and tasty.

Head for somewhere that makes it easy for you to control your choices. A sandwich, sushi, or noodle shop may be a better bet than a pizza or burger joint. But if your willpower can resist the pull of french fries, fast-food outlets are increasingly offering healthier options, such as salads or baguette sandwiches. If you know in advance where you are going, look online; most outlets often give nutritional information on their websites.

Whether or not you have calorie information to guide you, try to stick to healthy food choices from the menu, such as:

- Sandwiches with vegetables and lean protein, rather than fillings that are higher in saturated fats and mayonnaise.

- A salad on the side, rather than chips or fries.

- Meats that are grilled, rather than battered and deep-fried.

- Tomato- and vegetable-based sauces, rather than creamy and cheese-based ones.

- Extra portions of fruits and vegetables in side dishes and salads.

- Whole-grain varieties of breads, rice, and pasta, whenever possible.

- Fruit salad or sorbet, if you're having dessert.

- The "daily specials"—often freshly made from whatever is in season, and can make a tasty change from restaurant staples.

Putting healthy dining-out swaps into practice

INSTEAD OF	CHOOSE	BECAUSE
BLT sandwich	Smoked salmon and watercress sandwich	The unhealthy saturated fats in the bacon are replaced by healthy omega-3 fats in the salmon. Watercress provides vitamin C and calcium, and research suggests it may help reduce cancer risk.
Meatball panini	Roast chicken and tomato panini	Saturated fat is reduced by 7 grams per portion.
Standard main course salad	Order the same salad but with a dressing of lemon juice and no croutons	Adding lemon juice or balsamic vinegar to a salad instead of a cream or oil-based dressing saves about 200 calories—and removing the croutons saves another 200 calories. Don't be afraid to ask: most good restaurants are more than willing to oblige.
Spaghetti carbonara	Seafood linguine	Switching from the creamy sauce can save 300 calories a portion; a further benefit is extra zinc and iodine in the seafood.

TRY TO AVOID:

- Processed meats such as sausages and burgers.

- Lunchtime drinking, which can make you drowsy. If you do imbibe, minimize the effect by adding sparkling or soda water, or a low-calorie mixer.

- Creamy desserts and cheesecakes.

PERFECT PICNICS

Sunny days and warm weather tempt us outdoors for a different kind of lunch, but traditional picnic foods, such as fried chicken and cold-cut sandwiches, are often laden with fat and salt. Instead, why not take a little time to put together some healthy picnic treats, selecting from the vibrant array of fresh summer produce? Here are some ideas:

- Pull out the soft center of a large ciabatta loaf and replace it with roasted peppers, zucchini, and eggplant, with a dash of olive oil and a few chopped fresh herbs.

- Quiches don't have to be stodgy. Make your own using half whole-grain and half white flour for the pastry. Fill with plenty of vegetables.

- Tabbouleh makes a delicious, healthy picnic salad. Place the bulgur wheat in a small pan, cover with water, and boil for ten minutes, or as directed on the packaging. Add chopped parsley, mint, tomatoes, and red onion, and flavor with lemon juice and olive oil.

- Make a salsa. Combine diced tomatoes, avocado, red onion, a little finely chopped garlic, and chili (fresh, dried, or ground), then add a sprinkle of ground coriander or cumin, chopped fresh coriander, some diced mango or red pepper, and some cooked black-eyed peas for extra protein.

Just like everyday packed lunches, picnics need to be kept cool to ensure the ingredients are fresh and safe to eat. Use a purpose-made cooler with freezer packs or frozen juice cartons. Add ice to flasks of cold drinks, and avoid leaving your picnic in a hot car for too long.

Once outdoors, keep the food in the shade and covered until you are ready to eat. Take an antibacterial gel or hand wipes, and at the end of the day dispose of any leftover perishable food that has warmed up.

Chapter 22

DINNERTIME

Whatever time we eat it, our last meal of the day is often the one we enjoy most as we relax in the evening after work or play. Dinner can range from a stimulating social and family meal to being so tired we simply eat and slump in an armchair while watching TV. Tempting as that can be, it's not a recipe for good health. Nor is regularly eating a large meal late at night, at which point there's little time to digest it or burn off the calories consumed.

PLANNING AHEAD

It takes a little effort to eat healthily every evening, but planning menus and shopping is time well spent. It gives an opportunity to think about the variety of foods and nutrients in your diet overall. It helps you avoid buying more food than you need, saving you money and cutting out waste. Perhaps the greatest benefit of all is it helps the week run more smoothly, reducing at least one area of potential daily stress.

First, find a system that works best for you. Some people like to plan in advance precisely what they will eat each day of the week and follow set recipes; others prefer a more free-flowing approach that depends on what is in the fridge and how much time they have available. If you're cooking for a family on a busy schedule and depend on one big weekly shopping trip, the more structured approach can be the easiest.

You may need to ask yourself the following sorts of questions:

- What's already in the fridge that needs using up?

- What's in the freezer? If there are key staples in there, like chicken or salmon, work them into your menu plan.

- Where is everyone this week? When will the family be home together, and when will you need food ready at different times?

- Which days are you going to be most pressed for time?

- Who can help cook and take charge on certain days?

As you plan, try to keep in mind the balance of foods on the Eatwell Plate (see page 96), and at each meal include:

- Good-quality lean protein (fish, turkey, lamb, beef, pork, eggs, beans, and legumes).

- Plenty of vegetables (fresh, frozen, and occasionally canned) for their fiber, vitamins, minerals, and other plant nutrients.

- Starchy carbohydrates (potatoes, sweet potatoes, pasta, rice, and noodles). Use whole-grain products wherever possible.

Dessert is not essential every night, but it is an opportunity to increase the amount of fruit in the diet and to include a portion of dairy (just be sure to check the sugar content of low-fat products). At dinner, you should also:

- Eat at least one portion a week of oily fish such as salmon, fresh mackerel, trout, or tuna.

- Eat regular portions of nuts and seeds.

- Experiment with new recipes. It doesn't need to take hours or be overly complicated, but trying something new one night a week will help fend off menu fatigue. It can also help you to build up a repertoire of quick, tasty, easy-to-cook meals.

- Avoid eating processed meats too frequently. Bacon and chorizo are best used occasionally and in small amounts to add flavor to other dishes, such as stews and soups.

Between three and four hours before bedtime is the best time to eat your evening meal to avoid digestive problems that can keep you awake. If you are hungry at bedtime, a small snack combining carbohydrates and protein, such as a glass of milk with a banana or a multigrain cracker, can encourage sleep.

HEALTHY MEALS IN MINUTES

Some days, time pressures make it harder than usual to provide a healthy evening meal. Try these time-saving ideas for super-fast suppers:

- **Anything-goes, stir-fry saviors—**Stir-fry thin strips of meat or fish and set aside. Finely chop some vegetables, garlic, and ginger, and cook in the same pan for a couple of minutes, then tip the meat or fish back in for a final warm through. Season and serve with egg or rice noodles, which cook in 5 minutes or less.

- **Fish suppers—**Soft, white fish such as halibut and flounder can be grilled in minutes. Add extra flavor with lemon and parsley, pesto, or other toppings.

- **"No-cook" suppers—**With cooked chicken from a deli, you can whip up a quick Caesar salad. Put crispy iceberg or romaine lettuce in a bowl, cut the chicken into bite-size pieces, and toss onto the lettuce with a few ready-made croutons, plus some anchovies if you like. Top with Parmesan shavings and a drizzle of low-fat Caesar dressing, and serve with a fresh, whole-grain roll. Experiment with different ingredients and recipes.

Dinner for one

People are living alone in ever-increasing numbers, which means that many of us are cooking for one. It has advantages—you can eat what and when you like, regardless of other people's preferences or routines. On the other hand, it can be hard to drum up the motivation to cook a nutritious meal.

There can be practical difficulties, too. Most recipes are designed to serve four so must be cut down, although you may be able to save some for the next day or freeze it for a later date. Some cookbooks and websites specialize in single servings, so it's worth seeking these out or looking online.

Many supermarkets now stock single prewrapped portions of meat and fish, plus prepared meals and soups in smaller sizes. Better still, buy loose (unpackaged) fresh food, so you can have any size or quantity you like. A local butcher will be happy to provide single servings, and you can usually select how much fresh produce you need.

Here are some easy and delicious ideas for main courses and desserts for one:

• Grilled lamb chops with baba ghanoush—Cut an eggplant in half lengthwise, sprinkle with olive oil and black pepper, and roast it. Then scoop out the soft flesh and mash it with a teaspoon of tahini, crushed garlic, and juice of half a lemon. Grill two lamb chops under a hot grill, then squeeze the juice from the other half of lemon on them, and enjoy. Any leftover baba ghanoush makes a tasty lunch with toasted pita bread.

• Roasted fillet of trout and new potatoes—Put baby new potatoes in a baking pan with a little olive oil, and roast for 15 to 20 minutes. Add cherry tomatoes, artichokes, and the trout fillet, and roast for a further 15 minutes. Sprinkle with shredded basil and balsamic vinegar before enjoying.

• Baked figs—Set fresh figs in a small baking dish, cut a cross into the top of each, and drizzle with honey. Just before they're done, sprinkle a crushed amaretto cookie on top.

- **Dress up a prepared meal**—Don't do this often, but supermarket prepared meals can help when things get hectic. Use them as a base, but reduce their total salt and fat and add nutrients by adding, for instance, extra steamed broccoli to broccoli and cheese soup, more kidney beans and chopped tomatoes to a ready-made chili, or extra veggie toppings to a pizza, like sun-dried tomatoes, mushrooms, or artichoke hearts, all served with a large, colorful side salad.

PANTRY MAIN COURSES

Using ingredients you already have in your pantry and homegrown herbs, you can also whip up delicious dishes such as the following:

- **Tomato-poached fish with basil**—Lightly fry chopped onion and garlic in olive oil. Add a can of chopped tomatoes, black olives, and your choice of fish—whitefish or canned tuna both work well. Season with black pepper and perhaps a little Tabasco or paprika, and simmer until the fish is cooked. Stir in fresh basil. Serve with baby potatoes (you can add these to the simmering mixture to cook before the fish, if you like) or with pasta, plus a vegetable or salad.

- **Risotto**—Soften onions, leeks, or spring onions with finely chopped garlic in a little olive oil and butter. Put stock in a separate pan to heat through. Add risotto rice to onions or leeks, and stir to coat the grains. Add the hot stock to the risotto pan a ladle at a time, allowing it to be absorbed before adding the next. Leftover cold meat or ham can be cut into small pieces and stirred into the rice toward the end of cooking, together with frozen peas or corn. Heat through and serve with grated Parmesan, fresh parsley, and a side salad.

CREATIVE CARBOHYDRATES

Stuck in a rut with baked potatoes and pasta? Try some of these alternatives for a tasty change:

Family favorites the healthy way

TRADITIONAL FAVORITE . . .	. . . WITH A HEALTHY TWIST
Spaghetti Bolognese Sneaking in some extra veggies to your Bolognese boosts nutrients and helps your money go further. Use good-quality, lean ground beef to reduce the saturated fat. At the end of cooking leave to settle for a few minutes and skim off any excess fat with a spoon.	Fry chopped onion, garlic, ground beef, and chopped mushrooms in a little olive oil. Add a couple of cans of plum tomatoes and tomato puree, and 3 or 4 large carrots, peeled and grated (they won't be noticed once it's cooked). Season with black pepper, dried oregano, and a couple of bay leaves, and simmer until cooked. Remove the bay leaves and serve with whole-grain spaghetti.
Fried chicken & fries Simply removing the skin from chicken and baking, rather than frying, halves its calories. Fries made with sweet potatoes add beta-carotene, vitamins C and E, plus minerals—potassium, manganese, and iron.	Skin the chicken, top it with lemon, garlic, and a little olive oil, and then bake in the oven. Cut sweet potatoes into wedges, coat with olive oil, and roast for 30 to 40 minutes. Serve with a vegetable such as peas, beans, or broccoli, or with a side salad.
Beef in red wine Traditionally, this rich French dish is made with onions, garlic, red wine, beef, and mushrooms. You can make it healthier by adding more vegetables; the added bulk means you can use a little less meat.	Prepare in the usual way but, for four people, add around 9 ounces each of baby carrots, parsnips, and mushrooms with the wine and a bouquet garni. About 30 minutes before the casserole is ready, stir in 7 ounces fresh or frozen broad beans. Serve with a sprinkling of fresh chopped parsley.

- **Sweet potatoes**—Scrub and rub with olive oil, then bake whole as an alternative to normal baked potatoes. Delicious with vegetable ratatouille.

- **Bulgur wheat or quinoa**—These protein-boosting grains are great alternatives to rice or couscous. Boil according to package instructions and use in salads, soups, and casseroles.

- **Brown rice, wild rice, and pearl barley**—Both brown and wild rice have a nuttier flavor, are more nutritious, and provide more fiber than white rice. Brown takes longer to cook but can be used in most rice dishes. Wild rice (technically a grass) can be added to white or brown rice, or used in salads. Pearl barley helps to thicken a soup and makes it healthier and heartier.

- **Beans and peas**—Canned beans and peas are convenient, but dried are cheaper. Both are good value and a nutritious way to bulk out meals. Try out recipes using chickpeas, butter beans, black-eyed peas, string beans, kidney beans, edamame (young soybeans), lentils, and split peas. Most dried beans need to be soaked overnight and precooked before they are added to stews. Some, like kidney beans, must be boiled for the first ten minutes of cooking to neutralize toxins. Check instructions on the packaging. Lentils cook fairly quickly without soaking. Here are two quick bean ideas:

  - Try edamame and borlotti beans in a salad with steamed green beans. Crumble on feta cheese, drizzle with lemon juice and honey, and finish with a sprinkling of poppy seeds.

  - Make your own super-quick hummus. With a hand blender, blend a can of chickpeas with a teaspoon of tahini paste, a drizzle of extra virgin olive oil, a clove of garlic, and a squeeze of lemon juice.

PEPPING UP VEGETABLES

In Western diets, vegetables are often an afterthought. With such a variety of delicious tastes to enjoy and so many vital nutrients, they are far too important to be ignored. If you think vegetables are boring, try pepping them up in one of the following ways:

- Squeeze a little lemon juice over spinach or zucchinis—a quick, simple way to enhance their flavor.

- Drizzle steamed broccoli with a little toasted sesame oil, a dash of soy sauce, and a sprinkling of sesame seeds.

- Add softly fried spring onions to carrots. Or stir-fry thin carrot sticks in a little oil, add 1 teaspoon of lemon juice, and garnish with mint or dill.

- Stir-fry quartered brussels sprouts with pine nuts.

PERFECT EVERYDAY DESSERTS

If you must cater to a sweet tooth, chocolate mousse isn't the answer. Nor is cheesecake; a typical serving of a supermarket product contains around half the recommended maximum daily intake of saturated fat. Try these quick-and-easy healthy treats instead.

DAIRY DELIGHTS

Low-fat dairy products, such as yogurt or sour cream, have more bone-building calcium than full-fat versions. Here are some more tips to keep in mind:

- Put some berries such as raspberries or blueberries in the bottom of a small dish, add creamy plain yogurt and top with roasted almonds.

- Try frozen yogurt, a good, low-fat, and tasty alternative to ice cream. Beware, though, that supermarket products are often high in sugar. To make your own: tip a quart tub of yogurt into a freezer-proof container and freeze for an hour. Remove and whip with a fork to break up the developing ice crystals, then put back in the freezer. Repeat two or three times until frozen.

- Make a healthy rice pudding. Many recipes use cream, but you can make tasty rice pudding using low-fat milk (or soy milk), lemon, and a little sugar. Top with a spoonful of fruit compote.

A FRUITY END

Experiment with the many types of fruit available. All contain important micronutrients that boost the immune system. Try these:

- Roast autumn fruits, such as pears, plums, and apples, with a splash of apple juice, a sprinkling of brown sugar, and chopped dried apricots and walnuts. Serve with a small dollop of low-fat mascarpone.

- Roasted pineapple: Peel a fresh pineapple with a sharp knife. Cut into wedges, discarding the woody core. Put on a baking sheet, top with a small pat of butter and a grated star anise, and roast until bronzed and slightly caramelized at the edges.

- Fresh mango sliced and served with a drizzle of honey and lime.

- Fruit crumbles and pies that are "deep fill" to get in extra fruit and without a pastry base to reduce calories and fat. Add oats and chopped walnuts to your crumble toppings.

COOKING FOR KIDS

If you are feeding children every day, you want them to eat the same foods as everyone else. To encourage them to try new flavors, the best approach is to offer a few different foods on the plate so they can leave some without a battle. The balance of foods and nutrients on the Eatwell Plate (see page 96) is suitable for children from the age of about two years, although portions will be smaller than for adults. Before the age of five, children may need a slightly different diet. This should include:

- Whole milk between the ages of one and two years, then whole or low-fat milk from two to five years. Skim milk does not provide as much vitamin A, which is important for the developing immune system.

- Small portions of calorie-dense foods, as children need more energy for growth but have small stomachs. Nuts, seeds, eggs, and sardines are better options as they supply healthy fats, as opposed to salty chips or fries and sugary cakes and cookies. (Whole nuts should not be given to children under the age of five because of the danger of choking.)

- Plenty of fruit and vegetables as snacks, as well as with meals. A portion for a child is about the size of his or her fist.

If you want to cook something special, make it colorful and fun. Here are a few ideas:

- **Macaroni cheese faces**—Make a simple macaroni cheese more enticing and healthy by adding green broccoli hair, cucumber eyes, and a smiley tomato mouth.

- **Pick-and-mix plates**—On a pretty plate, set out small portions of diced cheese, sliced cucumber, chopped tomato and avocado, crackers spread with cream cheese, a little pile of grapes or strawberries, some dried apple, and other tasty ingredients. It's a good way to use up leftovers, and the kids will feel they are getting a treat.

- **"Invisible" vegetables**—It's important to offer vegetables on the plate so children get used to having them, but if your child is picky about veggies, take the pressure off by whizzing vegetables into pasta sauces and adding extra toppings to pizza.

- **Melon boats**—Cut ripe cantaloupe or honeydew melon into wedges and remove the seeds; slice the fruit away from the skin and cut it into chunks, leaving it in its skin "boat," Orange slices on toothpicks can make sails, topped with a grape or half a strawberry for the crow's nest. Younger children will need supervising when they dismantle it.

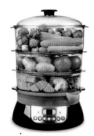

HOME ENTERTAINING

Inviting guests for dinner doesn't have to mean hours of stressful slaving in the kitchen producing soufflés, complicated main courses, and rich sauces. Don't be afraid to serve up simple, healthy dishes made with good-quality ingredients and bold flavors. You'll find your guests enjoy this just as much as fancy finishes. As always, planning ahead is crucial:

- Find out in advance if any of your guests are vegetarians or have a food intolerance or allergy.

- When and where can you shop? If possible make time to visit a good market, butcher, or fish store to get the best, freshest main ingredients.

- Plan courses that complement each other and the season. If you have a creamy curry or rich casserole, for example, cheesecake is too heavy for dessert. A rich main course requires only a light starter and dessert. Use fresh, seasonal produce when you can.

- Get your timing right—simpler food ready at a reasonable hour will go down far better than a flustered you serving elaborate dishes hours late.

- Don't panic if you get a bit behind. Set the table, light some candles, have some healthy nibbles and drinks ready, and no one will notice if it takes a little bit longer for dinner to arrive.

MAKING HEALTHY RESTAURANT CHOICES

In many ways, a healthy choice in a restaurant is much the same as a healthy choice at home: steamed or grilled rather than fried, especially deep-fried; boiled potatoes rather than fried or sautéed; tomato- or vegetable-based sauces rather than ones made with cheese or cream. The difference, though, is that at home you control the amount of ingredients like salt, cream, butter, and oil, while chefs often use these liberally. Their primary concern is not health but flavor.

Whether you need to worry about this really depends on how often you eat out. If, like many of us, you dine out only occasionally for a celebration or special treat, don't worry—your meal is meant to be enjoyable, not a source of anxiety. Go ahead and have a main course with a cream sauce; just have a fruit dessert or a sorbet instead of a rich cream dessert. If you eat out regularly, you should try to choose the healthier options.

Always be wary of the extras: the nibbles to start, the rolls with butter, the side order of fries, coffee with cream, the cheese plate, the after-dinner mints. Taken together, these can add up to almost a meal in themselves. Concentrate on your favorite courses. If you love savory foods, have a starter and main course but skip dessert. If you have a sweet tooth, leave out the starter. If you like all the courses, choose lighter options, or go for a second starter as your main, with a side of vegetables. You'll still enjoy all the different flavors and leave room for dessert.

Chapter
23

SPECIAL DIETS

Your teenage daughter announces, out of the blue, that she is now a vegetarian. Or your young son has been diagnosed as lactose intolerant and can't drink milk, which you know is so important for bone development. Or your mother who'd complained of thirst and tiredness has been told she has type 2 diabetes. Problems like this confront people all the time and require rethinking and changing normal everyday meals.

Special diets mean different food choices for medical and ethical reasons. They may mean avoiding particular foods or eating more of one type of food, but they should always supply all the nutrients required for good health.

If you have symptoms that you think may be linked to what you eat, it is worth consulting reliable websites, but make sure you take advice from a health professional. An immediate diagnosis may not be possible, but an initial discussion of symptoms with a qualified expert can indicate a sensible way to investigate possible links between food and not feeling good. In some cases, short-term trial-and-error diets can help confirm a diagnosis.

Seeking professional dietary advice is especially important for people who are more vulnerable to deficiencies, like fast-growing young children and teenagers. Pregnant women and people who are ill or recovering from illness also need expert nutritional guidance.

NOT EATING "FOOD WITH A FACE"

Even among those who still eat meat, an increasing number are choosing to eat less or have more meat-free meals. In the Western world, going one step further and becoming vegetarian is usually a health or ethical choice. By contrast, in countries such as India, millions of people are vegetarian for cultural and religious reasons, dating back to ancient times. In the West, most vegetarians follow a lacto-ovo vegetarian diet, not eating any kind of meat, poultry, fish, or shellfish, or products made from them (such as foods containing gelatin), while still eating eggs and dairy products. In India, eggs are often excluded, too.

Being vegan is a far more challenging and less-common dietary choice. As it cuts out all animal products from the diet—eggs, milk, and all dairy products, not just meat—it demands more radical changes in order to maintain a healthy balance of nutrients.

IS BEING VEGETARIAN HEALTHY?

Provided that you eat a variety of foods that are good sources of particular nutrients, a vegetarian diet is perfectly healthy. In fact, it actually seems to offer health benefits. Many large studies have found that, compared to meat-eaters, vegetarians are less likely to be obese and also seem to be better protected from heart disease and the risk of certain kinds of cancer. Almost by definition, vegetarians eat more plant-based foods, and this is linked to having higher intakes of fiber, antioxidants, and some vitamins and minerals. Also, vegetarian diets are usually lower in saturated fats, which are a risk factor for raised blood-cholesterol levels.

But these health benefits depend on vegetarians knowing what nutrients are essential for health and what foods provide them, then making sure that these are included in their everyday diet. A diet based principally on pasta and tomato sauce, for example—or on other starchy foods that are low in nutrients and high in sugars and salt—is not a healthy way to be vegetarian.

GETTING ENOUGH PROTEIN, VITAMINS, AND MINERALS

In most cases, vegetarian diets contain enough protein for good health (about 10 percent of calories), even though they're lower in protein than the diets of meat-eaters. Lacto-ovo vegetarians get protein from eggs and dairy products, and there are plenty of sources of plant-based protein—beans, lentils, nuts and seeds, soy, and other "meat substitute" products.

Vegetarians must also ensure they get adequate levels of all the necessary minerals and vitamins. Since they're usually taking in less iron than meat-eaters and because iron is less well absorbed from plant foods, vegans may not get enough. Adequate intake of calcium can also be a challenge for vegans.

Of the vitamins, B_{12} can only be found occurring naturally in animal-sourced foods, so vegans have to make sure that they eat products such as breakfast cereals that are fortified with

Vegan food sources of vital nutrients

Iron	Beans, peas, green leafy vegetables, dried fruit, and fortified foods (breakfast cereals, bread)
Calcium	Beans, almonds, green vegetables (kale, cabbage), and fortified foods (soy milk, tofu, bread)
Vitamin B_{12}	Fortified breakfast cereals, soy milk, rice milk, and yeast extract
Vitamin D	Fortified breakfast cereals, soy milk, soy cheese, and margarine
Protein	Beans and lentils, nuts and seeds, soy products, cereals, and meat substitutes

Seven foods for a healthy vegetarian diet

- Beans and lentils—in soups, stews, casseroles, curries, and salads

- Whole grains—in bread, pasta, breakfast cereals, pancakes, rice, and side dishes

- Leafy greens and other vegetables—in main and side dishes, soups, and salads

- Fresh and dried fruit—as snacks, in desserts, or in savory dishes

- Nuts—in salads, roasts, croquettes, cakes, puddings, or healthy snacks

- Milk and dairy products (yogurt, cheese) or soy-based alternatives

- Eggs

this vitamin (or take supplements); vegetarians usually get their quota of B_{12} from dairy foods and eggs. Although vitamin D comes mainly from the action of sunlight on skin, vegetarians, especially vegans, may not get enough from food. Again, vitamin D–fortified foods and supplements are helpful.

DIET FOR DIABETES: NOT SO SWEET

Insulin is the hormone needed to transfer glucose from the blood to the muscles, liver, and other tissues. Having diabetes means your body doesn't produce enough insulin or cannot use it effectively. If your diabetes is not identified and treated, carbohydrates in your diet cause glucose to build up to very high levels in the blood, which will make you excessively thirsty.

The condition also means that too little glucose gets transferred to the muscles, making you feel tired and weak. The aim of treatment—whether through diet, insulin, or drugs—is to keep blood-glucose levels within a narrow normal range, avoiding both hyperglycemia (high levels of blood glucose) and hypoglycemia (low levels of blood glucose).

There are two types of diabetes:

- **Type 1 diabetes,** which used to be known as insulin-dependent diabetes, occurs when the body cannot produce insulin and requires lifelong insulin injections to match the amounts of carbohydrates eaten.

- **Type 2 diabetes** used to be known as adult-onset diabetes, but today many young people are also developing the disease. It is caused by an insulin deficiency or insensitivity to the insulin made by the body, and is often linked to being overweight. Drug treatments can either increase the production of insulin or enhance its effectiveness, but weight reduction and control of carbohydrates are central to managing the disease.

THE "WHAT" AND "WHEN" OF EATING CARBOHYDRATES

While people with diabetes should eat a normal, balanced diet, the extra hurdle is learning "glycemic control"—how to balance the glucose-raising effects of eating carbohydrates with the glucose-lowering effects of insulin injections or hypoglycemic drugs. Foods high in protein or fat have little effect on blood-glucose levels, but eating too much can lead to becoming overweight, which is a high risk factor for type 2 diabetes. Too much saturated fat also increases the risk of raised blood-cholesterol levels, which are linked to cardiovascular disease. However, when planning daily meals and snacks, if you have either type of diabetes, you'll need to be especially aware of what carbohydrates you are eating and when.

You should be able to achieve normal glucose levels with

carbohydrate intakes ranging from 45 percent to 60 percent of total energy. Here's how to work it out:

1 gram of carbohydrate = 4 calories

45 to 60 percent of calories = 225 to 300 grams of carbohydrates (based on a daily diet of 2,000 calories)

Within this range, individual fine-tuning depends on the type and timing of insulin or medication, and on factors such as levels of activity and the type of carbohydrate.

If you are on fixed dosages of insulin at specific times of the day, you'll need a daily plan of carbohydrate intake timed to match the action of the insulin. If not, monitor your blood glucose and adjust your insulin intake to match the variations you find. It may take a while to balance insulin and carbohydrates to achieve long-term blood-glucose control; your dietitian will be able to help. If you're using insulin, make sure you have access to "emergency" carbohydrate snacks to counter possible episodes of feeling weak and shaky due to very low levels of blood glucose (hypoglycemia).

You'll need to learn about the glycemic effect of foods—that is, the rate at which they increase blood-glucose levels, as measured by the glycemic index (GI). Some carbohydrate foods, such as whole-grain cereals, beans, and many vegetables, are described as "low GI" because they cause blood glucose to increase only slowly after eating. Others, such as potatoes, white bread, fruit juices, and sweets, are "high GI" because they cause a rapid rise in blood glucose. Contrary to what you may think, sweet foods are not always higher GI than starchy foods.

CAN DIABETICS EAT SWEET FOODS?

The short answer to this is yes—in moderation. If you're diabetic, you can consume some sugar-containing foods, as long as most carbohydrates your diet come from starchy, preferably high-fiber foods. The use of calorie-free sweeteners does not affect blood-glucose levels. Nutritive sweeteners (such as fructose or sorbitol) have some effect, though, and consuming too much of them can also cause diarrhea or flatulence.

NO GLUTEN FOR ONE-IN-A-HUNDRED

Around 1 percent of adults in North America have an intolerance to gluten, a protein found in wheat, barley, and rye that causes celiac (pronounced SEE-lee-ak) disease. For people affected, eating foods containing gluten provokes an autoimmune reaction in which the body's immune system attacks its own tissues. The damage is done to the lining of the gut, so food is poorly digested, reducing the absorption of nutrients. Left untreated, the disease can lead to malnutrition.

The symptoms of celiac disease can vary widely between people, but usual problems are indigestion, feeling bloated, and diarrhea. Sufferers often feel unwell or lethargic after eating, and may experience unintended weight loss. There

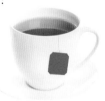

are many possible diagnoses for these general symptoms, so confirmation tests are needed to be sure that the trigger is gluten. Blood tests to identify heightened levels of tTG (tissue transglutaminase), an enzyme produced by damaged gut cells, is a reliable predictor of celiac disease, while a biopsy showing damage to the gut is the "gold standard" method of diagnosis.

Treatment for celiac disease is effective and simple: eat no gluten. But if you are diagnosed, you'll soon discover that what is simple in theory can prove difficult in the real world of restaurants, cafeterias, and everyday life. Foods may not be clearly labeled, and family and friends who cook for you may not be completely aware of what "gluten-free" implies. Treatment must also be lifelong, so that means saying good-bye to wheat or rye-based bread—although gluten-free pastas and pizzas are now widely available at supermarkets.

A GLUTEN-FREE LIFE

When planning a gluten-free diet, you must first become familiar with the huge variety of healthy, nutrient-rich foods that can be eaten. The good news is that most natural foods are fine—fresh fruit and vegetables, meat and fish, beans and lentils, nuts and seeds. Just make sure they have not been battered, sauced, or otherwise prepared with ingredients containing gluten. Rice and potatoes are gluten-free, and can fill the gap in starchy foods, or try buckwheat or millet for a change. Cornmeal, rice flour, potato flour, or chickpea flour can take the place of staple wheat flour.

Processed foods present more of a challenge. Some of the "do-not-eats" are fairly obvious: no bread, cookies, doughnuts, scones, cakes, pasta, pizza, or most breakfast cereals. Avoiding these is a start, but it's not enough, as very small quantities of wheat, barley, or rye are in many foods, often as components of other ingredients. Studying food labels will reveal surprising examples of "hidden" gluten ingredients, so label-reading is an essential skill that must be mastered.

IS A FOOD SUITABLE FOR MY GLUTEN-FREE DIET?

The first thing to look for is a gluten-free logo or statement on the label. Many stores have "free-from" food sections, which almost always include gluten-free items.

The next check is the ingredients list—is there any hint of a wheat, barley, or rye component in the food? Sometimes it is difficult to decide, because components of an ingredient such as "spice mix" may contain small quantities of wheat flour.

The final check is for "allergen alert" boxes. The presence of an ingredient containing gluten is one of fourteen food categories that most manufacturers now declare outside the ingredient list. Allergy-alert information is not a legal requirement, but it is quite common on food labels today.

Recent years have seen a dramatic increase in the number of products labeled fully and often specifically as gluten-free, so being diagnosed with celiac disease is less of a burden today than it might have been in the past. And you can always ensure that food is gluten-free when you buy and cook your own fresh ingredients. If you are diagnosed, you might also be advised to take multivitamin supplements because at times you may not be absorbing enough of certain nutrients.

ADVERSE REACTIONS TO FOOD

Sometimes, however much you like a food, when you eat it you experience a range of unpleasant symptoms. It may be difficult to establish if a food reaction is to blame and if so, which food is the culprit.

Adverse reactions to food are labeled as either a food intolerance or a food allergy. An intolerance is not a dislike; generally it means a physical adverse reaction to a particular

14 foods known to cause allergic or intolerant reactions

- Celery
- Cereal grains containing gluten
- Crustaceans
- Eggs
- Fish
- Lupin (lupin flour)
- Milk (lactose)
- Mollusks
- Mustard
- Peanuts
- Sesame
- Soybeans
- Sulfur dioxide and sulfites
- Tree nuts (e.g., almonds, cashews, walnuts)

food or ingredient that occurs every time you encounter it. Food allergy is a specific kind of food intolerance, where the food sparks an abnormal, sometimes dangerous, immune response in the body.

Although celiac disease is the dominant form of wheat intolerance, some people who are not celiacs experience persistent gastrointestinal symptoms that don't occur when they avoid wheat. Wheat sensitivity is difficult to diagnose, and the temporary exclusion of wheat-based products from the diet is often the practical way of establishing whether it is linked to the symptoms.

WHEN MILK ISN'T GOOD FOR YOU

The most common form of adverse reaction to milk and other dairy foods is lactose intolerance. To digest milk the gut must break down milk sugar (lactose), and to do that an enzyme known as lactase is required. Levels of lactase are high in the guts of infants, for whom milk is their only food, but in most adults, levels of this enzyme are much lower. When large amounts of milk are consumed, the lactose cannot be absorbed and passes undigested into the colon. Here, it gets fermented by gut bacteria, producing symptoms of bloating, gut pain, and diarrhea.

Lactose intolerance can be diagnosed with a hydrogen breath test. As symptoms depend on the amount of lactose consumed, you will usually be advised simply to reduce the amount of milk and fresh dairy foods you consume, although it may be necessary to exclude them altogether. The tiny amounts present in hard cheese do not seem to cause adverse reactions.

Infants and very young children can also be allergic to the protein in milk from cows, goats, or sheep. This can affect the gut (producing symptoms such as vomiting and diarrhea), the skin (atopic eczema, dermatitis), and the respiratory system (wheezing, rhinitis). Once the allergy is diagnosed, all dairy products must be avoided. Some children "outgrow" the allergy, and by the time they reach school age, milk may no longer produce the adverse symptoms.

PROBLEMS WITH NUTS

Peanut and nut allergies are less common, but reactions to even the smallest amount of nut can be severe. Symptoms can include urticaria (skin rash) and asthma. Extreme reactions can be life threatening, causing shock and swelling of the tongue and throat. People diagnosed with these allergies must ensure they eat nothing containing peanuts or tree nuts such as almonds, cashews, or walnuts. Although they may be allergic to one or the other, the advice is often to avoid both.

One ingredient to look out for is peanut oil, sometimes called groundnut oil, in cakes and sauces. Check food labels carefully. Peanut oil is also used in many Chinese, Thai, and Indonesian, and some West African meals, so these are "high risk" areas where you must make sure that dishes are peanut-free. Research suggests that peanut allergies, which are more common, occur more often in children and tree nut allergies in adults.

EFFECTIVE WEIGHT CONTROL

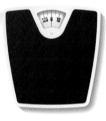

More of us are getting fatter every year. At its simplest, extra weight places strain on your joints, heart, and lungs. At a more complex level, excess fat can cause an imbalance in your body's biochemistry, now linked to a number of serious disorders including type 2 diabetes, high blood pressure, heart disease, stroke, and certain cancers.

With weight gain, your risk of psychological issues such as poor self-esteem and depression increases, as does infertility and impotence, and problems sleeping, breathing, and, in extreme cases, just moving. Exercise becomes more difficult, and the sheer pleasure of physical activity is often lost. The bottom line is that being overweight increases the chances of suffering poor health and having a lower quality of life. But it doesn't have to be that way. If you're determined, weight—however great—can be controlled.

IDENTIFYING A WEIGHT PROBLEM

A good starting point for assessing your weight is the body mass index, or BMI—a measure of how heavy you are relative to your height, used widely by the medical profession.

The BMI is a calculation of weight in kilograms divided by the square of height in meters (weight ÷ [height × height]). To take an example of a person 1.7 meters (5 feet 7 inches) tall who weighs 68 kilos (150 pounds): 1.7 × 1.7 = 2.89. and 68 ÷ 2.89 = 23.5. Using the chart at left, a BMI of 23.5 lies within the healthy range of 18.5 to 24.9.

The BMI adult weight guide

Underweight
Less than 18.5

Healthy weight
18.5–24.9

Overweight: 25–29.9

Obese I: 30–34.9

Obese II (severely obese): 35–39.9

Obese III (morbidly obese): 40 or higher

The BMI is a useful tool, but it can be misleading. A rugby player with a lot of muscle could be heavy relative to height without being overweight. Conversely, if you have a small frame, your BMI might fall in the healthy weight range while you're actually carrying too much fat.

Some variations come down to ethnicity. People of Asian heritage, for example, tend to be smaller-framed and carry more fat at a lower weight. There are also different BMI values for children because they have not yet fully developed.

HOW BIG IS YOUR WAIST?

The next step is to look at where unwanted fat is going. Fat stored just under the skin, called subcutaneous fat, and fat that accumulates on the thighs and buttocks is not such a health worry as abdominal (or visceral) fat around the organs. Build-up of visceral fat is linked to an increase in inflammatory chemicals in the body and to metabolic syndrome, a condition marked by high blood pressure and cholesterol.

To check if you have too much fat around your middle, measure your waist about half an inch above the navel and look at the list below; the lower measurements in the ranges are where doctors consider your risk begins. The higher your waist circumference and the higher your BMI, the greater your risk.

- **Men:** 37 to 40 inches or more

- **Women:** 31½ to 34½ inches or more

- **Asian men:** more than 35½ inches

- **Asian women:** more than 31½ inches

Half your height or less is the ideal waist measurement. Scientists have found that this simple calculation is just as reliable as the more complicated BMI:waist ratio for predicting future health risk.

GETTING READY FOR CHANGE

To achieve lasting weight loss and weight control, you have to really want to—and be determined to stick with it. Many people fail because they are not psychologically prepared for the challenges ahead. Thinking in advance about why you want to change, what it will mean, and what benefits it will bring can mean the difference between success and failure.

You'll also need to do some research and work out a strategy before you embark on your weight-loss plan. Identify potential difficulties and think of someone you can call on for support if necessary. When you start, be aware that some weeks will be harder than others, with less to show for it, and don't be shy of asking for help. To achieve long-term weight control, the changes you make to your diet and lifestyle must be sustainable.

KNOW YOUR DRIVERS FOR EATING

Are you someone who eats out of boredom? Or an emotional eater who uses food to cope with highs or lows? Do you eat from habit, while you watch TV? Or is your overeating social, or related to work and eating out with clients? Analyze where and why you eat to see what the problems are, then think about how you could reduce your calorie intake and increase your activity levels.

Different situations require different approaches. If you eat out of habit, find alternatives that do not involve food. Try knitting instead of snacking while watching TV, for instance. If it is social or work eating that is the root cause, make menu choices that fit with the food plan you decide to follow, be aware of portion sizes, and skip dessert. If you're an emotional eater, seek advice to help tackle more deep-rooted psychological issues.

GETTING INFORMATION

Family doctors may not give diet advice but can help you figure out your best starting point—whether you need specialist help from a dietitian, nutritionist, or psychologist, or if there are other medical issues that need investigation, such as diabetes or thyroid problems. If you want advice on food and diet, ask for a referral to a registered dietitian; when seeking nutrition advice, via your doctor or independently, it's important to consult a qualified professional.

Typically, dietitians do not give out prescriptive diet plans, but they do aim to guide you through decisions about food and answer practical questions. Some dietitians may be able to offer a regular point of contact to help keep you motivated, or recommend a weight-loss support group. A private registered nutritionist or dietitian can usually offer individual support.

OVERCOMING BARRIERS

Think about it: is there anything holding you back? For example, is lack of time or cooking skills getting in the way of eating healthily? Is the cost of food an issue? Does shift work dictate the times you can eat? Think of practical solutions.

Finding out about easily prepared healthy foods and learning some simple recipes to cook may be part of the answer. Shopping with friends for bulk bargains can help finances. Getting your partner or children involved can help, too, and lay the foundations for healthy family nutrition.

YOUR WEIGHT-LOSS STRATEGY

There's no magic to weight loss: despite all the different diets and thousands of words written on this subject, it comes down to the energy-balance equation. If you take in more energy (calories) in food and drink than you use, you'll gain weight; if you consume less than you use, you'll lose weight. So the options are: eat less, get more active, or—best of all—do a bit of both.

ENERGY IN—THREE STEPS TO HEALTHY EATING

Start with the basics of healthy eating; it may be all you need. The three things to consider are:

WHEN YOU EAT

Meal times are critical to healthy eating. People who "graze" erratically have been shown to eat more, not burn calories as effectively, have higher cholesterol, and produce more insulin than those who eat regular meals.

To balance your energy levels and keep cravings at bay, aim to eat every three to five hours, as this is the time it takes for the stomach to empty after an average balanced meal. Building in mini-meals in the form of healthy snacks helps keep hunger in check and prevents overeating at the next main meal. Timings for a typical day might be: breakfast between 7 and 8 a.m., a snack at 11 a.m., lunch at 1 p.m., another snack between 4 and 5 p.m., and dinner between 7 and 8 p.m.

WHAT YOU EAT

To supply all the nutrients you need, your diet must strike the right balance between the three major food groups: proteins, carbohydrates, and fruits and vegetables (plus some dairy products). You'll need some fat for good health, but not sugar, although a little sweetness can help combat food cravings.

- Proteins are essential to fuel growth and maintain, repair, and replace tissue in your body. Protein is also digested slowly, keeping you feeling full for longer, so for lasting satisfaction, eat some protein with all meals. You can get protein from animal or plant sources, although some non-animal sources may need to be combined—such as rice and beans—to give you a "complete" protein.

- Carbohydrates are an energy store for plant foods, and they are the same for us. Eating low-GI carbohydrates, such as whole-grain foods, keeps energy levels steady for longer, as they are digested slowly, and also supplies fiber to boost a sluggish gut and prevent constipation.

- Fruits and vegetables are perfect for piling on the plate because, with a few exceptions, they are low in calories but packed with protective nutrients—fiber, vitamins, minerals, antioxidants, and microchemicals.

HOW MUCH YOU EAT

Many of us pile too much food on our plates, and too often, it's the wrong kind of food. An easy way to portion food for weight loss is to start with a smaller plate—a medium-size (8-inch) plate is ideal. Fill half with salad and vegetables, then split the other half visually with a quarter for your protein choice and a quarter for carbohydrates—about two tablespoons of rice, potato, or pasta, or a slice or two of bread. The plate should look full, which is visually satisfying, and the food should take time to chew and eat, which helps you feel full.

ENERGY OUT—EXERCISE AND ACTIVITY

Diet alone can only take you so far before the body's metabolic rate slows down to compensate for getting less food. To lose weight and keep it off, you've got to get up and move. One U.S. study found that, on top of a reduced-calorie diet, you need an hour of exercise five days a week to lose 10 percent of weight and keep it off.

To increase your metabolic rate and burn off more energy, you have to get your heart pumping and build up your muscles; muscle is an active tissue, which burns energy even when it's doing nothing. Aerobic activity will raise your heart and lung rate, while weight lifting or resistance training builds and strengthens muscles.

At least thirty minutes of exercise should be a regular part of every day, so find activities you enjoy. Dance, swim, play tennis, or walk the dog. Use the stairs rather than the elevator at work to strengthen your leg muscles. Never sit still for long periods; get up every half hour. You don't have to go to a gym, but structured, guided exercise classes could introduce you to new activities and help you push your fitness to new limits.

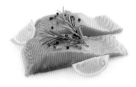

DIETS—FIND ONE THAT WORKS FOR YOU

Popular diets usually hit the headlines with some catchy angle that makes them sound fresh and new. Here's a closer look at some of them.

"FIVE AND TWO" FASTING

One of the most recently fashionable diets, the "Five and Two" eating plan involves two days of fasting in a week of otherwise normal eating. One 2011 study compared a regular weight-loss diet that reduced daily calories by 25 percent with the weight-loss results achieved by following a normal healthy diet five days a week, then a very low-calorie diet of just 600 calories on the other two days. Although some participants reported low energy, headaches, and constipation, those who stuck to the plan without bingeing on normal days lost as much weight as people on the daily diet. If this pattern suits you, rather than restricting calories every day, this could be a useful way to lose weight.

LOW-CARBOHYDRATE PLANS

These restrict carbohydrates (rice, pasta, grains, fruits, and some vegetables) to unnaturally low levels. The main food supply is protein (meats, fish, poultry, eggs) and fats. Treat foods (cakes, biscuits, chips, chips) are strictly off-limits—a key reason why the plans work. The diets all produce rapid initial weight loss, in part from water, so are effective in the short term. Protein is good for keeping you feeling full, so if plenty of meat with salad on the side is to your taste, this may be an easy type of diet to follow. No problems have been reported, but concerns have been raised about potential future effects on health.

LOW GI DIETS

These diets cut out carbohydrates with a high GI (white breads, sugary and refined cereals, potatoes, white rice, candy) and replace them with smaller portions of low-GI carbs, such as oats, brown basmati rice, whole-grain pasta and noodles, baby new potatoes, whole-grain pita and other breads, lentils, and beans. A low GI diet doesn't produce rapid weight loss, but works for some because it is easy to maintain long term as part of a standard, healthy eating-and-exercise plan. Essentially, it's a normal, healthy diet with a few small adjustments.

CALORIE COUNTING

Keeping a food diary, noting everything you eat and drink, has been found to raise awareness of the little things that add up. It's easy to do and worth a try to help you self-diagnose where you could make simple changes. There are cell-phone and online apps designed to help keep a daily log and calculate the details. They can be useful, but there is a danger of users obsessing too much over calorie detail while missing the basics of healthy eating.

WEIGHT-LOSS GROUPS

Commercial weight-loss groups such as Weight Watchers have good success rates. The weekly meetings help motivate, inform, and encourage dieters, and are a place to build community support and learn about healthy eating. The weekly weigh-in provides a timed goal for everyone to work toward.

VERY LOW-CALORIE REGIMES

These are the most restrictive of all, based on 800 calories a day (or less) from shakes or meal replacements. They are very tough to follow, but do produce rapid, short-term weight loss. If you would like to attempt a very low-calorie diet, you must discuss it with your doctor before starting and be monitored throughout. The daily shakes must include a good supply of protein to help limit muscle loss. Very restrictive diets are not recommended for everyone and should not be followed for longer than twelve weeks. However, for some, they are an effective weight-loss solution.

MONITORING AND MAINTAINING WEIGHT LOSS

Weighing yourself regularly—once a week, always at the same time of day—will help you keep track of progress, but it only gives you part of the picture. Muscle weighs more than fat, so if you are exercising and shaping up, you may not lose weight as quickly as you expect. Fluid levels may also change your weight significantly from one day to the next.

Well-fitting clothes with a fixed waistband can provide a good reference point: take note of how they loosen or tighten in different places. Once a month, measure your mid-upper arm, bust or chest, waist, hips, upper thigh, and make a note so you can track how your body is changing over time.

WHAT RATE SHOULD I AIM FOR?

The figures quoted for a safe rate of weight loss are usually between 2 and 3 pounds a week, but everyone is different. For some, weight loss is faster in the early weeks, then slows down as the body adjusts to changes in the diet. In practice, weight loss tends to follow a step-like pattern, rather than a straight downward line, with plateaus and occasional rises, too. If the overall trend is down, you know you are on the right track.

Set yourself upper and lower boundaries to allow for fluctuations, then adjust downward as you lose weight. Or use body measurements or clothes as markers.

If you hit a plateau but know you are following a good routine, don't panic. An occasional leveling off is normal and eventually will indicate that you've reached your ideal weight. But if a plateau persists while you're still overweight or if you start to cross an upper boundary, check for bad habits—diet deviations or less exercise, perhaps—and adjust your regime accordingly.

The same upper-and-lower-boundary technique works equally well for maintaining your target weight once you reach it. The key is to monitor yourself regularly: if you notice a weight increase, think about what has changed in your lifestyle to cause it and take small simple actions to get back on track.

INDEX

grains. *See* cereals; whole grains
heart health
    alcohol and, 51, 52, 93–94
    eggs and, 84
    harmful foods, 30, 33, 36, 42–43
    protective foods, 41, 58, 62, 69, 86
high blood pressure, 36, 51, 52, 80, 105
high-fructose corn syrup, 16, 36–37
hummus, 139
hydration, 45, 89–94, 141
hydrogenation, 32
infertility, 33
juices, 91–92, 129, 131
kiwi fruits, 62
lactose intolerance, 177–178
leafy greens, 63
leftovers, 120–122, 147
legumes (beans), 63–64, 139, 162
life stages, 73, 102–106
low-carb diets, 28
low-fat diets, 28, 75–76
lunch
    benefits of, 144
    for children and teens, 150–152
    at home, 145–146
    picnics, 154–155
    in restaurants, 152–154
    at work, 146–149
meat and poultry
    cooking, 119
    intake guidelines, 97
    processed, 41–43, 128–129, 154
    as protein source, 82–83
    seasonal, 109
mental health, 33, 51, 71
middle age, 104–106
milk. *See* dairy products
monounsaturated fats (MUFAS), 77–78
nighttime eating, 142–143
nut allergies, 137, 178
nuts and seeds, 62, 78, 136–137, 139, 149
obesity, 10, 33, 36, 40–41, 70–71
older age, 73, 106, 133
olive oil, 79–80
olives, 139
omega fatty acids, 32–33, 78–79, 87
onion family, 63
organic foods, 23, 30, 109–110
osteoporosis, 61, 84, 104
picnics, 154–155
polyunsaturated fats (PUFAS), 78
popcorn, 140
portion sizes, 21, 95–97, 184–185
potatoes, 97, 128
pregnancy, 62, 104
preservatives, 49–50

pretzels, 140
processed foods
    as addictive, 10–13
    described, 38–39
    obesity link, 40–41
    types, 15–17, 41–46
processed meats, 41–43, 128–129, 154
protein
    described, 81–82, 184
    intake guidelines, 97
    types and sources, 82–85
    vegetarian sources, 86–88, 170–171
    restaurant meals, 152–154, 166–167
resveratrol, 94
salads, 21, 145
salt, 47–48, 105
sandwiches, 46, 148
saturated fat, 29, 30–31, 76
seasonal foods, 108–109, 118
shopping, 107–113
smoothies, 44–45, 135
snacks
    danger zones, 137–143
    guidelines, 133, 134–137
    life stages and, 132–133
soft drinks, 35, 90–91, 151
soups and stews, 120, 121–122, 146
soy products, 15, 87, 130–131
spreads, 126–127, 137
stroke risk, 30, 33, 36, 51, 62, 105
sugars, 16, 34–37, 44
sweet potatoes, 149, 161
tea, 90, 129, 130, 174
thirst, 141. *See also* hydration
trans fats, 15, 29, 31–33, 76
vegan diets, 169, 170
vegetable chips, 45
vegetables. *See* fruits and vegetables
vegetarian diets, 86–88, 169–171
vitamin and mineral waters, 45
vitamins, minerals, 59, 60, 64, 87–88
water, 45, 89–94, 141
weight management
    maintenance of, 188–189
    preparing for, 181–183
    strategies for, 183–188
    weight guidelines, 180–181
whole grains. *See also* cereals
    benefits of, 41
    choices in, 42, 126, 134–135, 149, 151, 161–162
    intake guidelines, 97
wine, 92–94
yogurt, 85, 129
yogurt drinks, 131, 135–136
yogurt, frozen, 46
young adults, 103–104

Also Available from Reader's Digest

The most useful information in a most useful format, from the people who have been getting to the heart of the matter for almost 100 years.

The Reader's Digest Quintessential Guides— The Best Advice, Straight to the Point!

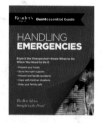

Expect the Unexpected—Know What to Do When You Need to Do It

- Prevent and handle accidents
- Cope with medical situations
- Quick repairs you can do yourself
- Stock the right supplies
- Keep your family safe

$14.99 • Concealed Spiral • 978-1-62145-248-5

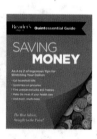

An A to Z of Ingenious Tips for Stretching Your Dollars

- Cut household bills
- Spend less on groceries (and eat better!)
- Find unexpected sales and freebies
- Make the most of your health care
- And much more!

$14.99 • Concealed Spiral • 978-1-62145-248-5

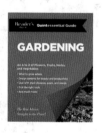

An A to Z of Flowers, Fruits, Herbs, and Vegetables

- What to grow where
- Design gardens for beauty and productivity
- Deal with plant diseases, pests, and weeds
- Pick the right tools
- And much more!

$14.99 • Concealed Spiral • 978-1-62145-291-1

Reader's digest

For more information, visit us at RDTradePublishing.com.
E-book editions are also available.

Reader's Digest books can be purchased through retail and online bookstores.